BED NO. 1

From Coma to Cycling:
The Resilient Recovery of a Covid Survivor

Laurence Penn

Published in 2025 by Author's Pen, 1 Fir Villas, Southwater Street, Southwater. RH13 9BN: www.authorspen.co.uk

© Laurence Penn 2025
The author's moral rights have been asserted

First published 2025

The right of Laurence Penn to be identified as the author of this work has been asserted in accordance with sections 77 and 78 of the Copyright, Designs and Patents Act 1988. This book is sold subject to the condition that it shall not, by way of trade or otherwise, be lent, re-sold, hired out or otherwise circulated without the publisher's prior consent in any form, binding or cover other than that in which it is published and without a similar condition including this condition being imposed on the subsequent purchaser. No part of this publication may be reproduced, stored in a retrieval system or transmitted in any form or by any means, electronic, mechanical, photocopying, recording or otherwise, without the prior permission of Author's Pen, its publishers.

British Library Cataloguing in Publication Data available
ISBN 978-1-8383436-7-5 – paperback
ISBN 978-1-8383436-8-2 – e-book

We were unable to contact the copyright holder for the timeline on pages 220-221. If notified the publisher will be pleased to rectify this omission at the earliest opportunity.

Printed by Ingram Spark, Milton Keynes, Buckinghamshire.
Edited and proofread by Author's Pen
Typesetting by Helen Jones
Cover design by More Visual ©MoreVisual

To my hero ... Martine

BED NO. 1

Foreword

It's just over five years since the world experienced the COVID pandemic. Personal accounts are important to bear witness to a period of tragedy and suffering. But they also help to remind us of the countless acts of kindness, during a time when people came together to help others.

For two years people in our hospital, like healthcare workers in countries across the globe, became accustomed to the repetitive presentations, the downhill trajectories and, for the lucky ones, the slow often painful recoveries. Laurence, in bed one, was one of many, but as his book powerfully recounts, each had their own background, scared families at home and collective struggles to survive.

I found reading the book at times harrowing, funny, uplifting and cathartic. It's a story of one person's experience of deteriorating to being as close to death as possible, before painfully inching back to health. After displaying courage to recover we then see the desire to give back something, to say thanks and help others who experience critical illness. The recovery journey from critical illness is a long one. But as Laurence describes, with determination and help from others, it can be traversed.

Dr Luke Hodgson

Intensive Care and Respiratory Consultant at University Hospitals Sussex NHS Foundation Trust and Honorary Clinical Reader at BSMS

BED NO. 1

Thanks and acknowledgements

Martine, Yasmine and Mischa for your love and unwavering support.

All my family (Sue, Rachel, Julie, Alannah, Saskia)

Dr Tim Fooks, High Sheriff of West Sussex for his incredible knowledge and insight, for decoding the NHS acronyms and language into facts my wife could understand and for always having space for me on some epic Gryphon adventures.

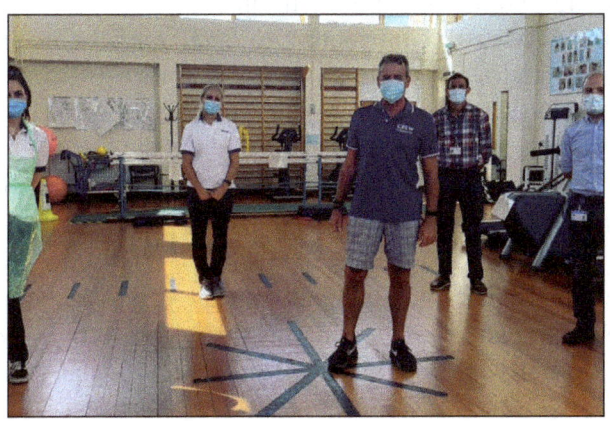

Figure 1

Amelia Palmer, Respiratory and Intensive Care Physiotherapy Lead, Worthing Hospital,

Western Sussex NHS Foundation Trust ... I am proud to call Amelia and Rick friends. Amelia truly went above and beyond in caring for me and getting involved in my quest to generate interest in my recovery and the cycle across the South Downs Way (SDW). And of course, the book, *Bed Number One*, getting the team together so they could be interviewed – you are truly an amazing human being.

Tom and Ruth Simmonds, for their unwavering love and support and, yeah, for Tom doing the SDW challenge with me.

Dr Luke Hodgson, one of the kindest and most unassuming heroes I have ever had the pleasure to meet. Thank you for agreeing to get behind *Bed Number One*. Luke, I'm looking forward to making the research utilising smartwatch tech/ Fitbit a reality across the NHS.

Dr Todd Leckie, he may have been responsible for planting the cycling idea in my head, I have a vague memory of talking to him about his triathlon exploits!

Sam Morfee, for contributing to *Bed Number One* and for being such a lovely person.

Grace Dowding, always making me laugh. And I'm sorry recruitment made you cry.

Mary Kate Standing, such positivity, always made me feel energised! Thank you for agreeing to be part of *Bed Number One*.

Gemma Stoner, mostly thank you for your care, you were just amazing and I know you may think you were *just doing your job* but your genuine love and care for what you do is awesome.

John Price, Special Projects Fundraiser, My University Hospitals Sussex. What an epic gent, supporting me through the early stages of the entire plan to ride SDW and for being a constant supporter of *Bed Number One*, the charity are very lucky to have you.

To all the wonderful nurses who met me at the halfway point in Storrington – what an inspiration you all are, x.

Linda Folkes, Clinical Trials Nurse/ Research Champion Lead, thank you for being so involved in *Bed Number One*. For being an awesome leader of the research champions and an all-round, super human being.

Heather Fox, thank you for contributing to *Bed Number One* and for your friendship. A real pleasure getting to know you.

To all the Sussex Research Champions: Lou Goodhall, Maddy Bell, Ann Bates, Alan Sutton, Dave Chuter, Simon Porges, Melissa Day, Caroline Humphreys, Lara Tozer.

Annelieke Driessen, Qualitative Research Fellow/ Ethnographer University of Oxford

Honorary assistant professor, London School of Hygiene and Tropical Medicine, intensive care and Covid study.

Lucy Ainsworth, Programme Officer of Nursing and Midwifery Office, CRN National Coordinating Centre (CRNCC), National Institute for Health Research (NIHR), for looking after me before during and after all the *Nursing Times* awards, will never forget that – brilliant!

Karen Wright, Senior Quality Manager, Infection Prevention and Control Workstream.

Samantha Wallace, Principal Speech and Language Therapist – Clinical lead for H&N and Voice Disorders Service.

Adrian Dessent, Patient and Public Involvement and Engagement (PPIE) Manager, LCRN Kent, Surrey and Sussex Core Team, NIHR Clinical Research Network (CRN), who first enrolled me as Research Champion.

Dr Andi Skilton, Senior Manager for Public Engagement and Involvement, CRN National Coordinating Centre (CRNCC), NIHR Clinical Research Network (CRN).

Jackie Condliff, NIHR public engagement team, UPH CRNCC.

Beth Allen, Senior Manager: Impact, Intelligence, Engagement and PPIE, Department of Health & Social Care.

Professor Nick Lemoine, Medical Director, Executive Team, NIHR Clinical Research Network (CRN).

Mike Wood, brilliant cycling and fitness advice and friendship and SDW companion.

Alex Merricks for brilliant support throughout the SDW ride on the day

All the wonderful people of Thakeham, especially the gin aficionados.

To all the exceptionally generous people who donated to the JustGiving page – truly awesome!

Malcolm Shaw and ITV, for getting behind the story and bringing it to life. The help from ITV has been and continues to be awesome, superbly supporting local news and local causes.

Paul Clark for his generosity and financial support.

Cover Design, Richie, via Author's Pen, for the inspired cover design @MoreVisual Ltd.

Helen Jones, typesetter via Author's Pen, thanks for making this book fly.

Author's Pen – Lesley Hart – brilliant work and quite literally could not have done this without your patience and guidance.

Ted Gooda, via Author's Pen, thank you for the website design – looks amazing.

To the many awesome unnamed NHS people who nursed me back to life and to health – I may have been a motionless body lying in bed number one but you all cared for me and many others in a way that goes so far beyond *doing the job*. The love you have for life, for the NHS, for the human race – thank you all so very much.

And YOU … thank you for buying this book.

Thanks and acknowledgements

BED NO. 1

Contents

Foreword	v
Thanks and acknowledgements	vii
Chapter 1 A meeting to remember	17
Chapter 2 Hospital landing	29
Chapter 3 ICU	33
Chapter 4 Martine tries to make head or tail of it	39
Chapter 5 Guarded in Groundhog Day	55
Chapter 6 A change of scene	60
Chapter 7 Critical	67
Chapter 8 Research trials and tribulations	74
Chapter 9 Hope and help	81
Chapter 10 Separation and steroids	88
Chapter 11 Bright lights, prayers and Richard Hammond	92
Chapter 12 Martine and reality	100
Chapter 13 Delirium, delusion and FaceTiming	107
Chapter 14 Ta-da!	119
Chapter 15 One step at a time	123
Chapter 16 The imaginary toilet and other stories	128
Chapter 17 The famous four on the third floor	133
Chapter 18 I would know that fully PPE protected person anywhere	139
Chapter 19 Are we nearly there yet?	148
Chapter 20 Home is where the hard work is	152
Chapter 21 My second-best bed	155
Chapter 22 Two sits down, one stand up	162
Chapter 23 A bit Fitbit	167

Chapter 24 Cornwall and heart	174
Chapter 25 Training	180
Chapter 26 We're putting you on the board	190
Chapter 27 Research champions	193
Chapter 28 The South up and Downs Way	200
Chapter 29 Every end is a new beginning	206
Appendices – The clinical view of events and some data provided by the NHS	217
List of images	222
Glossary	226
About the author	239
Notes on contributors	240
One last thing before you go	243
Bed Number One – fundraising	244

Contents

BED NO. 1

Chapter 1
A meeting to remember

I was tempted to start my story with the intense darkness, with the vivid coma dreams, with the bright light, the prayers, the space man's hat, or even with my constant companion – the travelling bed – but no. To make any sense at all, I will have to launch off from the beginning. In contrast, the commencement seems rather ordinary, hardly something to hook you in. The setting was a mundane meeting room. One that was warm and unoccupied, which is why I nabbed it while it was free.

Normally I would be sat in an open plan office, but hidden away in that meeting room I wasn't being accosted by well-meaning colleagues sidling up with, "Laurence, could I just have a minute?" or "Laurence, quick question …" and "Laurence, can we just discuss *such-and-such*?" I could get some work done, gloriously undisturbed. Or so it seemed. I set myself up with my laptop open, my phone boasting good signal and the satisfying knowledge that after one more appointment I would be settled for the rest of the day.

I had come from a board meeting to discuss whether we would need to shut down the business, put employees on furlough and even face the risk of redundancy. There were a lot of numbers coming at us: 118,000 cases across 114 countries and as of the 11th March 2020: 4,291 deaths. The most recent news reported an outbreak at a ski resort at Ischgl in Austria. It seemed the revellers there had spread Coronavirus particles all over Europe. This *thing* that had shut down parts of China was really on the move and God only knew where it was now.

I entered the warm, cosy, contained room, with the express intention of having a meeting with an employee. As soon as he walked in, I could tell something wasn't quite right. He sat across the table from me, sweating buckets and kept wiping his brow. It seems funny now, doesn't it? I had come from discussing hundreds of thousands of people getting sick, to looking into the exhausted, sickly eyes of this guy and I didn't think, hey, I wonder if there's a connection. Call it optimism if you will, but for some reason it just didn't occur to me. What I did was tell him he looked rough. I actually said, "You look shit, mate. Go home."

He thanked me and made a hasty exit. Good for him. He really hadn't looked at all well[1] and had just got back from a trip to somewhere in Africa. We were all at it then, travelling far and wide for business. I'd been to Dubai twice already that year – in late January and early February. Dubai is such a massive international hub, there were people coming and going from who knows where. Could I have come into contact with the new coronavirus there? The first cases of COVID-19 outside mainland China were confirmed in Japan, South Korea, Thailand and the US as early as 20th January 2020, it is not beyond the realms of the imagination that it might have also been in Dubai by then.

*

Approximately a week after my afternoon in the cosy, contained, meeting room, we made the business decision, that everyone would work from home. UK Prime Minister Boris Johnson had begun his daily press briefings. The UK

---

[1] Incredibly he was not hospitalised but became unwell.

death toll was up to fifty-five. It was during the third week in March. I had been feeling fine.

I had always been fit. Done at least two circuit training classes a week. I love mountain biking and I used to teach jiu-jitsu. I was in good shape, always had been. Anytime I did feel out of sorts, I would put it down to travelling. Getting to the office to spend time with the team involved a soul-crushing commute every day: three hours of drive time going there and coming back. Working from home put a stop to all that. I had to rely on Zoom or MS Teams to hold meetings and keep up to date with the sales guys but I quite enjoyed it to be honest. Without the commute I had extra time in the morning and evening. What a bonus! Maybe I could get used to this.

That weekend, I went out for a walk with my wife. We were on the South Downs, near where we live. The sun was shining and there was that hopeful vibe of spring. We took the very steep chalky path. A real lung buster of a climb with amazing views of Sussex and the sea. It's about a five-mile loop and at the end there is a little coffee shop in a converted barn. The perfect stop for great cakes and a steaming cup of coffee but today wasn't going to be a walk like any other.

I just remember thinking, God this is hard, much harder than it is normally. I was wrestling with myself about not feeling great – not really feeling myself – but I didn't twig. I am an eternal optimist so pushed the nagging doubt to the back of my mind. We got the coffee and cake to go.

When we got back home, I did something I never normally do. I lay down on the floor. It was in the lounge. I didn't even make it as far as the sofa.

Martine, my wife, asked if I was OK. It wasn't like me to lie down.

"Yeah, I just need five minutes," I said. And I went to sleep right there on the carpet.

*

"The TV was like a constant companion, always there, feeding us a never-ending stream of fear. I hated how it never stopped. How it was always there, haunting the background of our lives. I told Loz, 'We have to turn it off.' But he insisted, 'I need to know. I need to hear what's happening.'

One morning, despite my plea, the news was on again. There was a report from Italy, and I couldn't turn away. The footage was haunting. A woman was slumped against a hospital wall, her body shaking with sobs. Her husband had just been admitted to hospital. I couldn't look away, even as my heart broke for her.

I stood there, tray in hand, and watched – frozen. The weight of her grief pressed down on me. Later, I felt it. That tightening in my throat. My breath caught. *That's weird,* I thought. But I didn't really think Loz had COVID-19. It didn't make sense, not at that moment. So, I pushed the thought away." *Martine Penn*

*

It was a strange feeling coming down with COVID-19, like you were being pulled under. Things that should have been easy suddenly weren't. Even standing felt too much like hard work. I *had* to lie down. At some point I made it from the lounge floor into bed – with a startlingly exhausting climb up the stairs.

The next day the symptoms really kicked in. I started to feel much more uncomfortable: very hot, then cold, then hot, with the beginnings of a little tickly, irritating cough. Despite my seemingly constant attempts to shift it, the cough wouldn't clear. It kept on itching. I was coughing and coughing and coughing. I became a really irritable person because I was so angry with this persistent scratchy feeling lodged in my throat.

I was gulping flu powder, like nobody's business. Martine was going out, I said to her, "Can you get me some paracetamol?"

Many shops were closing; people were struggling to get certain items. In the supermarkets whole shelves were being cleared: Bread, tinned food, dried pasta. It turned out people were panic buying paracetamol too. It was one of the few things suggested for fighting this mysterious illness. And as no one knew how it spread, hand sanitiser was also in very short supply. A bit harder to understand was the rush on toilet paper. Martine worried about not being able to get paracetamol. We were running dangerously low.

It was then Martine got a phone call from one of our daughters. Mischa had been working for a recruitment company in London. Her employers said everyone needed to work from home, so she went from being in an office five days a week to sitting on a laptop on her own. For Mischa that also meant working from the confines of a flat share where she was renting. London was becoming a ghost town, with rumours that whatever this illness was could mean six months of isolation. People who remained in the city were in their own little worlds, rushing about, but Mischa felt there was a rising panic. She didn't want to get stuck in London, so she talked to Martine about an exit plan and packed up her things in a day.

"Oh, my goodness, talk about panic packing! I was shoving everything in. I left half of my belongings behind, literally tossing stuff into a bin. Amazing what you can do in a hurry." *Mischa Penn*

As they were texting the arrangements, Mischa asked how things were at home. 'What was going on?' she typed.

Martine sugar coated it. Well, she would; she's a mum. She replied, 'Yeah, well, I think Dad's not very … he's got a cold. Looks to be a bit of a nasty cold but nothing to worry about."

My daughter and her partner had been quite unwell back in February but had no way of knowing what illness that might have been, so it was still daunting for Mischa to walk into this house of sickness. Everyone was imagining I would be fine. I would fight it off in a few days, wouldn't I? It is true, I can struggle with colds. Due to an operation I had well over twenty years ago to remove a growth next to my lung: a nerve (phrenic) that controls the diaphragm had to be sacrificed which means my left side lung and diaphragm are a little less effective at shifting a chesty cough or cold, so unbeknownst to me the family was worrying about me more than they let on. Would this aggressive new virus kick my butt?

Martine told me she was driving to London to get Mischa. On the way back they managed to find a huge, well-stocked supermarket where they picked up some essentials … like the bog roll. Martine had tried her best but even in the large supermarket, instead of paracetamol, she had to buy cold and flu drugs, the ones stuffed full of caffeine. I was thinking, I can't sleep; I need to sleep and you're giving me caffeine! Without even knowing it, I was giving her a hard time. But in my head, I thought, I just need some paracetamol and I will be fine.

The limited sleep meant I was getting confused. If you have ever had a really high fever, you will know you have these strange erratic and panicky dreams that fitfully come and go and you are not quite sure if you are dreaming or you are awake. Trying to watch the news was no help. I was in a muddled state of not feeling good, struggling to breathe comfortably and I couldn't see any end to it. The news didn't seem to see an end to it either.

Mischa remembers, when she got home, I was bedridden and pretty unwell.

"It was all a whirlwind to be honest. Mum was obviously very stressed about the fact that everything could go into lockdown, 'Do we have enough food?' or 'Is the rest of our family alright?' And for me it was like: Oh, God, I need to sort my life out. What am I doing? I was still working, so I had my full-time job going on in the midst of it.

I was trying to look after Dad at the same time. Mum said, 'Right, you can't see him. You've got to leave stuff at the door. He's staying in the bedroom,' so I actually saw him from across the hall. I only came in occasionally to give him a cup of tea, but he'd just stay in bed. It was odd because I *couldn't* really see him, and he obviously wasn't himself. Horrendous fevers, so he's obviously not feeling like he wants to have a nice conversation either, which is fair."
Mischa Penn

Talking was increasingly difficult because the coughing started to become a real chore. Were my lungs shutting down? It felt really awkward and difficult to do anything. Even going to the toilet presented a struggle. But I was convinced in my head I was getting better. I was sat in bed, fully clothed, wearing a big ski jacket, wrapped in a duvet with the heating on and I was still cold. But surely, I was getting better?

"It was a bit of an odd time. Everyone was in a bit of a blip, weren't they? I think Dad was feeling it too. Dad's very good at putting on a brave face. 'I'm fine,' even though he could be quite literally *dying*. He's like, 'No, I'm all good. OK.' I think at this time, though, when they don't say anything, you know, that means it's not good." *Mischa Penn*

*

I could see Martine and Mischa were worried about me. Martine wasn't sleeping in the same room. She had isolated me. Cottoned on. Even though, I still hadn't. She thought I had got COVID-19 but there were no tests at that time to prove her right. There wasn't even a very clear line on what the symptoms were. Nobody really knew *anything*.

Martine was packing a bag. And I was thinking, what's going on? I tried to remember. It was day seven of me trying to fight off a nasty flu with rest and paracetamol. It was not quite going to plan. Mischa and Martine were having conversations about calling for assistance.

"Loz had been isolated in our bedroom for a week, I was still taking food into the room. We knew it had to be COVID-19, it was impossible for it not to be. It was everywhere. On the TV, the radio, the newsfeeds. Relentlessly constant. The numbers climbing. People dying." *Martine Penn*

"Initially we were thinking, he'll be OK, we just need to stick it out, keep him well fed, and keep him hydrated. It got to a point where you thought, no, there's nothing that Ibuprofen can do, so let's call 111. We actually had quite a few conversations about it because we were obviously making him take his temperature and asking him about his breathing. This is when we were hearing all the stories of people dying – elderly people struggling to breathe.

We were on the phone trying to get through to 111 for hours. As you would expect it was a busy old line." *Mischa*

Penn

"Hello, Mr Penn?" a voice on the other end of the phone said. The phone seemed to have found its way into my hand quite suddenly.

"Yeah?"

"This is Dr Jones. Your wife has called 111 and I'm calling in response to that call. I need to ask you a few questions, OK?"

"Yeah." It would have been rude to say no and besides, it was starting to dawn on me I just might need a little help.

"Mr Penn, your wife has taken your temperature and you're forty degrees. Are you having trouble breathing?"

"Yeah." I coughed a lot then. Who was I kidding? Coughing was what I did now. *All* I did, it seemed.

"Can you hold your breath and count to ten?"

"Yeah …" I was confident I could. Such a simple ask. "One, two, three, four …" I was coughing again, spluttering all over the place. I had to change my answer. "No."

"Mr Penn, I've called an ambulance. Please be ready to go. I hope you get well soon."

"Thanks," I said. The die was cast.

Barely ten minutes later and an ambulance arrived at our house. I could see the blue lights strobing through the curtains. The voice of two paramedics carried through the hallway. Down the stairs I went, dressed like the Abominable Snowman. I was wearing a whole load of these jackets. I was thinking it will be all right, it will be all right; I will be OK.

I was at least in good company. The two paramedics were also amply dressed. Wearing their full personal protective equipment (PPE), they looked like they were in hazmat-style suits[2]. It was daunting and Martine and Mischa seemed

---

[2] Hazmat is an abbreviation of hazardous materials

quite freaked out by how they looked: hands covered, feet secured, paper-looking suits over their clothes and their faces protected with masks. It was like they had come to us from the Planet Zog.

"Yes, they turned up and I thought: Oh, am *I* supposed to look like this around *you*? I don't know if you've ever watched *Monsters Inc.*[3] but in that film they come in those white suits to take away the little contaminated sock; it was like that. They turned up kitted out in special gear to protect themselves. Obviously, you saw it all over the news, so you got used to it eventually, but the first time seeing it was a bit odd. It was like they'd taken away some weird, contaminated little thing." *Mischa Penn*

The paramedics immediately took my temperature and said, "Right, we've got to get off these clothes. You've got on too many. And you're over forty degrees. Your temperature's really high."

"But I'm cold," I said.

Mischa remembers how I was muddled.

"Very confused. His body wasn't focusing on thoughts at that point, it was focusing on trying to heal itself, on fighting off the bad bits of COVID-19, so he was struggling to put together sentences. *He* was obviously just focusing on the fact that he felt awful." *Mischa Penn*

The paramedics took the extra clothes off me. And I was just thinking, Oh, OK, maybe it's not so good then, maybe I've got it bad, whatever *it* is. Still, I didn't know what it was. I was starting to figure it might be COVID-19. I had been expecting it to be a bad flu that I would get over quick enough. I was still in denial but I could see the ambulance

---

3 2001 Pixar animation studios film for Walt Disney Studios also known as Monsters Incorporated.

crew didn't look happy. From within their beekeeper-like paraphernalia, they looked out with faces hanging heavy with concern.

The paramedics did a test where they put a clip on my finger. It measured the amount of oxygen in my blood, which showed them how well my lungs were working.

It was something like sixty per cent when it should have been at around ninety-eight per cent.

My wife gave them the bag and my iPhone. As I passed her going through the front door I tried to say, "I love you" and "See you soon," but ended up coughing in her face.

"I knew taking him to the hospital was the right thing to do. I knew that we couldn't do anymore to help him because obviously, if he is ill and he's got COVID-19, he needs medical care. No matter how much he was good at saying he was OK, it was almost like we had to tell him that this was the right decision. Watching him go away in an ambulance … it's a blank bit of emotion, because you don't know how to feel. You can't feel the emotion because nothing's technically happened yet. You assume he's going to come back. You don't assume he's not. You just think, the hospital is going to take care of him now, but I can't go and see him, so it was a bit of a weird goodbye. We hugged him, both of us also knowing we probably shouldn't have hugged him because he had COVID-19, but you can't *not* hug your dad, can you." *Mischa Penn*

They helped me into the ambulance, assisted me onto the bed where they put an IV line in me for fluids. They put me on oxygen too. Surely, that would help? It was a strange sensation; there was a hissing and a cold feeling. It had a taste, slightly metallic, though that may have been my taste buds stopping functioning.

I heard the medic say, "I don't like the look of this count. I'll get him strapped in and we need to get a shift on."

I was made to feel as comfortable as possible but I had never been in the back of an ambulance before. It was daunting. There was so much technical equipment. There was the paramedic, still in his hazmat-like suit, sitting on a swivel chair, working on me, chatting to me. He said, "OK, Mr Penn, it's going to be a bumpy ride but we'll get you to Worthing as soon as we can."

The ambulance lurched forward. I could sense the bumps and turns as we made our way out. I could sense the speed. I heard the siren go on, probably to get someone out of the way. There must have still been some souls out there on the lonely streets. It felt like the small hours of the morning – one o'clock, two o'clock – but it was evening. It was dark, the streets deserted due to the National Lockdown. It had begun five days before. Although, I had been so sick, I barely noticed it happen.

It was awkward without Martine with me. I kept feeling guilty because I knew she would be worrying about me. I was still thinking: Oh, they will sort this out in a few hours, get me breathing right, pop a few drugs in me, and I will be home, right as rain!

Out of the side of the skylights, I could see the blue lights flashing. We were really motoring along. I tried to map the route in my mind, trying to work out where we were turning, what roads we were on when we were going straight ahead.

The paramedics were talking again.

"Right, can you tell them to get something prepared? We're coming in the A&E[4] entrance and his oxygen is still low and falling."

---

[4] Accident and Emergency

Chapter 2
Hospital landing

Whoosh! The doors opened and more hazardous materials (hazmat) suited people dived in. They grabbed for the bed. One of the paramedics was still sitting beside me but his *spacecraft* had come to a stop and these new people were now dragging me out. I made to stand up but the whole team urged me against it.

"Oh no, you stay in bed Laurence."

As the bed moved out of the ambulance, wheeled legs sprung from the bottom. I was feeling very disorientated and delirious but I *did* know I was being pushed towards A&E at Worthing Hospital. I recognised it as I was propelled away from the ambulance. I tried to mumble a thank you to the paramedics but as I went to speak all that occurred was more coughing.

From the stretcher, I was aware of more voices, of seeing people's heads from a surreal angle. But mostly I saw ceiling, a whole lot of hospital ceiling.

They wheeled me into a cubicle in A&E. Many people talked to me, asking questions. They all wanted to know, "How do you feel?" And I tried really hard to tell them but I was still coughing.

A line was put in my arm for fluids. They took blood samples from my other arm. I was hooked up to several monitors, so my oxygen and heart rate could be closely monitored.

I did manage to get a quick photo of it all occurring. I

sent it to Martine through WhatsApp saying, "I'm OK, xx".
I didn't really look OK. Was I OK?

*

Time went by but I wasn't aware of day or night. In A&E the light is always on full. It is hard to get a sense of time. I was aware of reassuring words being uttered but it struck me I hadn't seen a smile for a while. How could I? Everyone's lower face was completely covered. A small sensation of fear bubbled up in the pit of my stomach. Was I in trouble here?

They put me on another oxygen device. There were constant tests. They were trying to work out what was going on. They were monitoring me very closely and maybe because of that I let up. I totally lost track. I don't know if I slept. I don't know what I did. I'm guessing I lay there and kept on with coughing and the attempts to breathe in the oxygen they were trying to pump into me.

It became a blur of comforting words, "Mr Penn, you're in Worthing A&E. We are looking after you. We're just going to give you *this, and that, and something or other*, to make you more comfortable."

And they did as they said, because over the next forty-eight hours there were times when I *was* feeling strangely rested and relaxed. It must have been the drugs because in reality I was struggling to cope. Was I just too stubborn to admit I was in a really bad way?

I was moved to the High Dependency Unit (HDU). There they propped me in a bed. I was wearing a very attractive, three-quarter length hospital gown. The lines in my wrist were still there, dispensing fluids and drugs. Like in A&E, it was busy. There were people around all the time. I got used to it, which is weird. It gave me a sense of security. I was being looked after. There was a nurse, continually at my bedside.

Senior consultants were closely monitoring and it was through them, I sensed they were still not happy with my oxygen count. The next thing I knew, I was wearing what appeared to be a dated spaceman's helmet. It went over my entire head and round my shoulders. The device was pumping out a hundred per cent oxygen in a desperate attempt to get it into my blood stream. The contraption felt uncomfortable and was noisy. A constant hissing sound, the pitch changed when I inhaled to when I exhaled. When I coughed it just went crazy.

I still hadn't shifted that non-productive dry cough. It kept on and on. I was absolutely knackered but the *nice* drugs had me thinking it was all very interesting. A continuous positive airway pressure (CPAP) hood? Specialist breathing apparatus? A space helmet? I was going to be fine. I thought this is obviously it; I'm going to get better now. This is the thing that will do it. I took a selfie and sent that to my wife to try and keep her in the loop: me in the space helmet. I wrote, *Love you*. The message said sent on 31st March 2020, so that must be it. Two days I had been in hospital. Three days? How could that be?

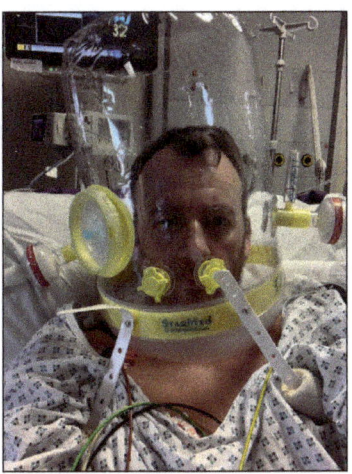

Figure 2

Well, I'll be out of here in no time now, I thought. I'll be home tomorrow. It'll be great.

Then my phone was taken away.

I was given medication in tablet form. I'm not sure what it was but it made me throw up inside the space helmet. Oh dear. It was taken off abruptly. Had I rejected my sci-fi prop? Surely, I needed it. The air out here wasn't going to sustain me. The atmosphere was too thin. Although it was quite a relief not to have the discomfort of the space helmet, I was painfully aware that it was my only way of surviving the hostile environment my body was rejecting. I wanted my space helmet back ... minus the vomit, if possible.

How long had I been here? *Was* it really three days? Had I slept? I started to get confused. I couldn't seem to think or function. I was feeling restless, anxious and exasperated. Something was happening, but what?

I overheard, "He's just not getting enough oxygen; we need to do ..."

What did they say? I couldn't hear. I had not slept ... maybe ... not until now ...

Chapter 3
ICU

My hospital admission notes say: 28th March 2020, 21:23, a fifty-four-year-old man was officially admitted to Worthing Hospital. He had a severely low oxygen count, shortness of breath, a high fever and a cough. He was otherwise an extremely fit, active man. Just over twenty-four hours later he was admitted to ICU as his condition declined.

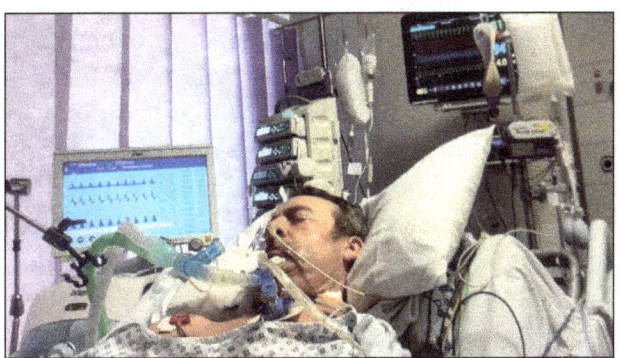

Figure 3

Dr Luke Hodgson, an Intensive Care Respiratory Consultant at Worthing Hospital, was the senior doctor in charge of the intensive care unit at the time the fifty-four-year-old man was admitted. This man in freefall decline was, of course, me – Laurence Penn, Loz to his friends – but Dr Luke Hodgson didn't know *me* yet. I was just some words on a form and a body lying in a bed, struggling increasingly to breathe. Luckily for me that kind of thing was in his wheelhouse.

Dr Hodgson knew a great deal about respiratory conditions, but what was new to him and his team, like all other healthcare professionals, politicians, policymakers, to me, to my wife, and to everyone else in the world, was COVID-19. This was not a day like any other in the *office*.

Along with his colleagues, Dr Hodgson had been watching the storm clouds gather over China. For a while it looked like the outbreak might be contained. However, humans will travel. Flights the world over continued to take off. Buses carried their fares across countries. Heavily populated trains traversed tracks. Personal vehicles sped from A to B to Z. Boats, ships and ferries still took holidaymakers on trips, tours and even cruises.

By 11th February 2020, the news had broken that of the eight confirmed cases in the UK, one was a healthcare professional who had worked a shift in Worthing A&E.[5] It had been an unnerving time for staff at the hospital. It suggested the inevitability of the march of the illness. A sliver of hope remained that COVID-19 might follow a similar path to previous illnesses that had failed to become as widespread as initially feared.

SARS, another coronavirus-based illness affecting the respiratory organ, saw an outbreak in 2003. It had travelled to two dozen countries in North America, South America, Europe and Asia but hadn't spread extensively within many countries. Globally a total of 8,098 people became ill with SARS, according to the World Health Organisation[6]. Of the eight in the United States, all had travelled to areas heavily affected by the illness. No spread was thought to have

---

[5] https://www.theguardian.com/world/2020/feb/11/uk-man-linked-several-coronavirus-cases-speaks-hospital-steve-walsh

[6] https://www.cdc.gov/sars/about/fs-sars.html

occurred in the local US community.

However, when the large outbreak of COVID-19 cases occurred in Northern Italy – the first locally transmitted hospitalisation was confirmed in Lombardy on 21st February 2020[7] – it became harder to deny the inevitability of the rapid spread of this particular coronavirus. Staff at Worthing Hospital went on calls with experts from China and Italy before any patients came forward because the understanding grew that as the days went on; the wave *was* coming.

They could see that in China, patients were put on ventilators rapidly. The outcomes were looking like hardly anyone was surviving when the illness got to that stage. For healthcare staff like Dr Luke Hodgson there were early indications that at the most severe end of the scale things were looking bleak. The Intensive Care Unit (ICU) team were forced to quickly assess what they were going to do if huge numbers of patients were suddenly admitted who were extremely ill.

When I was admitted to the ICU, I joined other patients who were battling this aggressive virus. Dr Hodgson remembers that, of the first severely ill patients admitted to Worthing Hospital with COVID-19, not everyone made it out the other side. Unbeknownst to me, I had joined the elite group of the ventilated. I was, however, living proof that the nature of this society was disputable. Healthcare professionals from nurses to doctors to the research team confirmed they struggled to understand the criteria for what enrolled each of us into this life and death dance with COVID-19.

During the first wave of the pandemic, the pressure on the ICU and High Dependency Unit (HDU) was immense.

---

7 https://www.theguardian.com/world/2020/may/29/why-was-lombardy-hit-harder-covid-19-than-italys-other-regions

Worthing Hospital being a District General, or non-specialist hospital, it is relatively small compared to other hospitals. Normally it would have six intensive care beds and six on the high dependency unit. Intensive care might be someone on a ventilator or a kidney machine. In contrast, a high dependency unit might involve someone being on support for blood pressure. Under COVID-19 conditions, the usual number of patients admitted doubled and then tripled. Whereas once they might have had a maximum of six patients ventilated at any one time, during the pandemic that went as high as twenty. They had to expand the area. ICU expanded into HDU and then into Cardiology.

Like many hospitals in the country, Worthing ordered extra ventilators as patients began to mount up. Ventilators essentially do all the work of a person's lungs. The problem was not just the quantity of critically ill patients needing them, but also the length of time they were expected to be on a ventilator. Compared to other serious illnesses that might require a patient to be on a ventilator for a matter of days, COVID-19 was seeing cases that required weeks.

Around the time I was admitted to hospital, breaking news whipped up the fear that a ventilator shortage was inevitable. America was stockpiling the machines and, in the UK, MP Matt Hancock set an extraordinary quota for manufacturing more of them. Various companies, some of which had no experience of producing ventilators, started working on these machines. As a result of the panic, a number of manufacturers went back to the drawing board, creating a brand-new ventilator prototype. Dyson was said to have been personally contacted by the PM and a group that included McClaren also got to work.[8] The ventilator saga

---

[8] https://www.theguardian.com/business/2020/may/04/the-inside-story-of-

would rumble on for some time and it was something that unnerved my wife. Would I be bumped off my ventilator if a more *deserving* case appeared?

However, it wasn't straightforward. Not everyone who became seriously ill with COVID-19 went on a ventilator. As Dr Luke explained, the practicalities surrounding the decision were more complicated. Like with any other severe medical illness, it is only people who are otherwise physically fit that can survive the intensive care treatments.

Your body is fighting the minute they plug you into that thing. For somebody who has underlying conditions – a heavy smoker, a heavy drinker – are they going to put that guy on the ventilator? There is much about being intubated that is gruelling for the body. Therefore, for someone who is already very fragile and frail going on a ventilator probably wouldn't be appropriate. Couple that with the initial evidence coming out of China: that if a patient needed to go on a ventilator, their likelihood of survival was very low. Therefore, the decision to put me on a ventilator was not one that was taken lightly. I was assessed as someone who was normally fit and active. When the ICU team had reviewed me in my still conscious, if somewhat confused, state they concluded that I seemed panicky but I said I was feeling OK, just very thirsty.

Studies have shown that in numerous cases COVID-19 caused the symptom of dry mouth[9]. It also turned out that my feeling OK may have been more than stubborn optimism. Dr Hodgson reflected on reports that some COVID-19 patients, despite severe problems with the lungs, entered a sort of happy hypoxia phase.

---

the-uks-nhs-coronavirus-ventilator-challenge

9 https://journals.sagepub.com/doi/pdf/10.1177/0145561320960353

This is something that has been speculated on since the first wave of the pandemic.[10] If true, it might mean that despite having very low oxygen levels, I could have seemed, from the end of the bed, to be relatively comfortable and doing OK, compared to an equivalent severe problem in another case, for instance a person with standard pneumonia. Some people, therefore, like me, despite being very unwell, might be talking and seemingly not looking too bad. In these cases, the severe problem can then create a seemingly rapid decline.

Much later I would meet another guy who was told he was about to be put on a ventilator. That must have been odd. He was given twenty-five minutes to call his wife to tell her he was going to be sedated. I didn't think I'd had that. My wife didn't know anything. Although she tried to ring, she didn't speak to a doctor until the next morning. They seemed surprised she didn't already know. Overnight, I had experienced increasing repository failure and was now in a coma.

---

10 https://www.science.org/doi/10.1126/science.368.6490.455

Chapter 4
Martine tries to make head or tail of it

After I'd been transported from home and into hospital, Martine and Mischa were left waiting for updates. You will remember, as soon as I had arrived at the hospital, I had texted my wife with my brand of positive spin but after the space helmet, silence had ensued. What must they have thought at home?

The phone call Martine received on 31st March 2020 informing her of my induced coma must have been a shock. If only this was an ill-judged foolish joke appearing one day too early. But no, I really was lying sedated in bed number one on the ICU Ward of Worthing Hospital. Dr Todd Leckie explained the deterioration in my lung function to Martine. I was critically unwell and the prognosis was difficult to predict. The doctors suggested I would likely need at least several days of ventilation. I was currently *critically stable.*

It had been recorded that I was informed about being intubated before it happened. Apparently, I requested Martine should not be contacted until the morning so she wouldn't be disturbed overnight. I don't remember any of this but it does sound like something I might say.

Dr Hodgson would later tell me how at times saving a patient's life just had to take priority over phone calls to their loved ones. This may have also been why the first thing Martine, waiting at home, knew about it was after I had already been put into the coma. Hospitals were having challenges adjusting to the new circumstances. At this time, like never before, once a person was admitted to hospital, they became closed off to the outside world.

Normally within hours of admission to intensive care, consultants like Dr Hodgson would be looking after the patient, giving the family updates in person at the bedside. The families would be involved, made aware of the severity of the condition, but this was a pandemic and very little was known about how COVID-19 spread. The strict no visitors' rules had to be observed. The hospital had zones for those infected by the virus. I was shut away behind multiple closed doors.

"Once Loz was placed into an induced coma in ICU, everything changed. I wasn't allowed to visit. I wasn't even allowed to call. At the time I needed to hear how he was more than I've ever needed anything. I was met with silence. Loz, unconscious and clinging to life, couldn't message or call. And I hadn't had the chance to tell him I loved him before they put him into an induced coma. So, I waited. For a phone call. At any time. Sometimes in the middle of the night, sometimes not at all. The waiting became its own kind of suffering: quiet, torturous, endless. I understood the reality: staff couldn't just stop everything, strip off their PPE and run to the phone. There wasn't enough PPE to spare. They were overwhelmed, under-resourced. Yet, they showed up day after day, fighting to keep people like Loz alive."
Martine Penn

"I think our hospital quite quickly made a fair bit of effort in terms of dialogue with relatives, because we know patient outcomes are better if you can actually get some interactions. And obviously for the family, things like PTSD are more likely if you've not had enough interaction … So, there were various efforts made to mitigate for the fact that people couldn't visit." *Dr Luke Hodgson*

Martine wasn't allowed to see me and hospital staff knew this could have an impact on treatment and recovery. Instead, she got daily phone call updates. Doctors found themselves in the difficult position of trying to communicate sensitive information to relatives from a distance. Martine remembers being enraged that a TV crew[11] were allowed into hospital but not her or relatives. Nonetheless, it was hard for NHS staff to put themselves in the shoes of these voices on the end of a line but they tried their best.

"When the consultants called, they were calm, composed and impossibly kind, despite the crushing pressure they faced. I could hear it in their voices, they were fighting for him. They knew he was strong, healthy, a father, a husband. I held on to that. I wanted every detail. I wanted to help. I wanted to do something. But all I could do was stay optimistic, hold myself together and thank them for every small act, every update, every hard decision they had to make.

I believed, completely, that they were doing everything humanly possible to save his life. All the while, much of the country was sat at home, complaining about boredom or arguing that COVID-19 wasn't even real. While I sat by my phone, praying. Waiting. Twice, they called to tell me I should prepare for the worst. That Loz might not survive the night. There are no words for that kind of helplessness. I managed somehow. To this day, I still don't know how.

I held it together, because I had to. For our daughters. For Loz. For myself. I clung to hope like it was oxygen, whispered prayers into the dark and made myself believe – really believe – that he would survive. That he'd come back

---

[11] Ross Kemp on the NHS Frontline, a twenty-four-minute documentary on Apple TV

to us. Then I'd try to sleep. Not the kind of sleep that rests your body, but the kind that tricks your mind into shutting off just long enough to escape the fear. I'd lie in bed listening for the phone, half expecting it to ring with the worst news, half willing it to stay silent.

Every morning, I woke up and checked I hadn't missed a call. Every night I went to bed with my heart in my throat. But I didn't fall apart. I couldn't. I built my strength in the cracks of the unknown. In the seconds after bad news. In the silence between updates. In the space where love and fear lived side by side. That's where I found something I didn't know I had. A kind of resilience that doesn't look like bravery it just looks like surviving.

The calls never stopped. Messages flooded in from family, friends, his GP, neighbours, work colleagues, even people we hadn't heard from in years. All asking the same question: How's Loz? Please keep me updated. And I did. I answered them, day after day. Summoning the strength to be the one who carried the weight of the bad news. Repeating the same words, trying to soften the blow without losing the truth. It was exhausting: mentally, emotionally, spiritually.

There were days I wanted to disappear. To escape the endless noise of media, of people's panic, of well-meaning concern that sometimes just reminded me how alone I felt. I wanted to sit in silence, just me and my horse, in the stillness of the stable. Somewhere the world didn't need answers from me. Somewhere I could breathe, without expectation. Having Mischa, my youngest daughter, at home was one of the things that held me upright. She's always been wise beyond her years, grounded, and stronger than most adults I know. Every day she showed up working from home, keeping to routines, staying calm. She didn't even tell her employer or her colleagues that her dad was in the ICU, fighting for his life. That quiet strength ... it was everything.

Yasmine, my eldest, carried her grief differently. She had to cope alone. Isolated from us. Still going into work every day as a key worker, putting on a brave face while her dad lay in a coma. I can't begin to imagine the loneliness she must've felt, the helplessness. None of us could be together but we were all holding the same pain." *Martine Penn*

*

Subsequent research has since revealed that, as Dr Hodgson alluded to above, a significant number of relatives suffered post-traumatic stress disorder (PTSD) as a result of not being able to see their loved ones.[12]

Daily phone calls kept a relative in the loop but this link was not without stress. Every relative had a different way of coping with the tension. Martine never knew when these calls would arrive, which must have added to her stress levels. By necessity, calls were at varying times of day depending, for example, on how I had been overnight or what actions had been taken or how I had responded to a certain course of drugs.

Luke Hodgson said of Martine, "Certainly I think her way of coping and trying to get through this was to try and be helpful, but also to get as much information as possible. Some families appear not to be fussed at all. They'll just take ten seconds and they don't want to know anything more. You have a spectrum of people. Some people want to know absolutely everything."

Martine was following the path of COVID-19 like a hawk. She had a vested interest and she didn't want to miss a thing

---

12 https://jamanetwork.com/journals/jama/fullarticle/2809191

that might help me in my desperate position. She wasted very little time. The following day she started out by using part of her phone call to ask about the anti-malarial treatment – hydroxychloroquine – which was being discussed on the news as a possible cure.[13] Dr Todd Leckie explained this was currently under investigation and not part of *standard management*.

Standard management wasn't too difficult a phrase to decipher but there was more code to come. Martine is a therapist; she has knowledge of health matters but some of the language used by the doctors was difficult even for her to fully understand. Mischa was with Martine during some of the phone calls from the hospital. They would put the call on speaker phone.

"My mother is the one person to find you a solution. She definitely made this process a lot easier for me, because she'd say, 'Look, it's going to be OK; this is the reason we'll be fine.'

She's doing research, speaking to everyone, speaking to all the doctors she could. We have a family friend who is also a local GP, who was very invested in helping because he's good friends with my dad. He's giving Mum every possible: 'Speak to them about this …' or, 'Ask them about this …' and, 'Make sure they do this …' etcetera. which actually, I think, helped a lot and also gave my mum some clarity or some comfort. She then understood the language that the doctors were using because they use all these different f***ing words. Do we understand them? Absolutely not. Dad's local GP friend was absolutely giving us some reassurance and saying, 'No, this is what this means …' and 'Yes, that's OK,

---

13 https://newsroom.uw.edu/news-releases/does-antimalarial-drug-prevent-covid-19-study-seeks-answers

…' or 'Those are normal, …' All that good stuff, so that was really, really helpful." *Mischa Penn*

"On Thursday, 16th April 2020, Ross Kemp aired a documentary about the NHS frontline, where he went inside an ICU to report on the impact of COVID-19. Watching it made me absolutely furious.

The ICU had told me, time and again, that there was a severe shortage of PPE, that they couldn't let me in because there wasn't enough protective equipment. For over two weeks, I hadn't seen Loz. And yet, here they were, letting Ross Kemp and his entire film crew walk in.

They said they had permission from the patients to film, to show the world how difficult things were for the staff. But I couldn't understand how that was even possible. How could they give a camera crew permission, but not me, his wife?

I was enraged. It felt so wrong. So unfair. It was as if my right to be with my husband was being denied, while a camera crew got to waltz right in. I felt completely powerless. I was so upset, angry, confused, betrayed. It wasn't just the contradiction, it was the raw pain of being kept away and yet seeing others allowed access in my place.

I had thought, deep down, that if Loz were to pass away, it would be a nurse holding his hand, not mine. I had prepared myself for that possibility, knowing I couldn't be there, but that thought: at least it would be someone kind, someone there with him, kept me going.

But they let a camera crew in. A group of strangers, with their cameras and their crew, allowed inside when I wasn't. The cruel irony of it hit me all at once. I wasn't allowed to hold my husband's hand during what could be his final moments, but they were letting people in to film for a documentary.

It felt like a punch in the chest. How could this be? How could that be the reality we were living in?

We were in full lockdown. Everything was closing and the rules were changing by the hour. It felt like the world was closing in around us. But if you had a dog, you could still walk it, so everyone was walking their dogs. It was surreal. There were these crazy rumours going around, they said, dogs and cats could spread COVID-19. It felt like nothing made sense anymore." *Martine Penn*

*

Martine's secret ally would help her navigate this unusual situation. This ally was our friend Dr Tim Fooks. We didn't know Tim in a professional capacity but his daughter and ours had been friends, which had led to our friendship. He proved to be a highly effective interpreter. Tim reflected on the relatives' position.

"It's very difficult, isn't it, to listen to something when your mind is actually just full of questions, uncertainties and emotional responses? And so, Martine did really well. She's obviously a highly capable, competent person, and she did really well to be able to handle as much information as she did. Even then, it's not at all surprising that there were things that were said to her, the consequences and the significance of which she couldn't be expected to fully understand." *Tim Fooks*

Martine was highly appreciative of the calls she received from the consultants but, as Tim put it, "Highly specialist people, whether they be doctors, engineers, military – whatever they do – have a language they talk in which is designed to be very precise but is also technical and allows you to short-circuit, perhaps, some of the big explanations, which are necessary for people who don't have that language."

Tim also added, "I understand what was useful for Martine was helping her understand what she was being told. To [grasp], therefore, what was happening to Laurence in a way that gave her understanding. Which meant that when she was then speaking to the consultant, she was able to understand enough to be able to engage with the conversation. It didn't make Laurence better, but it made it easier for her to cope with."

Aside from being a wonderful bloke, Tim had been a GP in Pulborough since 1992. He talked about how views in medicine changed in more recent years from a more patriarchal or authoritative manner of communicating with patients and relatives, to ways of explaining diagnoses and treatments so they can be fully understood. He acknowledged that this has accompanied a more general understanding of well-being and how our minds can affect illness.

During this extraordinary year, Tim stepped down from his practice to take up the post of High Sherriff of West Sussex, an appointment he was given by the late Queen Elizabeth II. His year as High Sherriff would have in a normal year been full of appointments but during 2020 it was a very different experience.

"I think it certainly was ironic that I was the first medic to ever be High Sheriff in West Sussex and the year I would be given this honour was the one that proved to be the COVID-19 pandemic." *Dr Tim Fooks*

Tim wrote articles supporting charities whose normal roots of communication had been severed and he organised a conference on loneliness. When he did eventually get back to his practice, what had happened to me affected how he viewed his work. He acknowledged that it seemed no one was quite safe from COVID-19, "… or could assume that they were safe from it. You couldn't rely on just generally being fit to protect you. Were you going to be the person who was going to be knocked out by it or sail through it?"

Tim had achieved his science degree in the middle of his medical training in 1984 at St Mary's Medical School, where penicillin was discovered by Fleming. St Mary's was at the centre of research at the beginning of the 80s for HIV, "Which is really the last pandemic that we've had, albeit one that affected more specific groups of people." Tim's specialism was infection and immunity. Studying viruses and bacteria, coronavirus was on the syllabus because twenty-five per cent of colds were caused by it.

Talking of COVID-19 he said, "It's not an unusual virus in terms of a new discovery but clearly this particular variant was very remarkable because of its quick transmissibility. Initially, as often happens when new viruses appear, it brings tremendous danger."

Due to his background, Tim would prove very helpful to Martine: this was a subject he was familiar with and able to comment on in view of having a scientific background, "And that was great. To be in a position where I could give her a little bit of insight, sometimes a lot of insight into what was happening so she was able to understand the significance of what people were saying to her."

Martine produced a list of areas where she needed to increase her understanding and Tim helped her by drawing on his medical knowledge. He said he was frustrated not to be able to do more to help me directly as I lay in the coma, but it was great to be able to help a friend indirectly as best he could. To get some idea of the medical terms and language being thrown at Martine, let us look at his explanation to me of how my immune system was combatting the virus.

"If you think of the immune system as a defence system (because that's what it is, it's not an attack system by definition, it's a defence system) then it is organised very much on a military sort of basis. So, it has systems that allow you to immediately respond to a range of different attacking particles, whether they be bacteria that sits on your skin and gets into a cut, or whether it's a virus that you inhale through your nose. It can remember what viruses or bacteria it's been exposed to and create a more rapid response to that particular particle on second exposure.

It organises the responses differently depending on what type of issue it's dealing with. There's what's called cellular immunity and there are antibody type immune responses and it has lymph nodes dotted around key parts of the body where infections are likely to get into the system, which act as fortresses: in which the defence systems can be both prime but also centred to ensure rapid deployment of protection near the area where the infection has come in. It's really remarkable ... You have a separate system for your gut than you do for the rest of the body.

When you get an infection, it's going to be dependent not just on what your natural immunity can do, but how big the inoculation by the virus is at the beginning. Your glancing blow on a pavement when someone just comes past with a few particles is very different than if you're standing by someone on a train who's coughing in your face. And of course, Laurence had a meeting with a work colleague where he spent half an hour or so with a really sick man in a closed environment. That man will have been shedding gallons of virus, so Laurence would have had a huge inoculation. It may be nothing more than that [why Laurence was so affected by COVID-19]. It's like an army. If you send in a million soldiers, it's going to be a very different battle than if you send in 10,000.

One of the key features to it, as it is with any defence system, is that you stop firing your weapons when the battle is over, because obviously, what happens if you carry on firing the weapons and deploying your troops? You're going to cause yourself damage. Therefore, quite a lot of the issues people have had with fighting any infection, not just the COVID-19 virus, are that the damage is being created by the response to the virus. And that is another factor that can determine whether someone will have been able to have an appropriate response that deals with the virus and effectively switches it off – the response stops it and it's all tidy – or whether there's a huge response to this virus.

Perhaps the person has been exposed to something similar in the past and they're now producing a huge response which doesn't stop. Or indeed its own attack is so vast that actually there's collateral damage that's created to tissues that have been affected, or to the surrounding areas.

I'm certain Laurence had a huge inoculation of the virus at the beginning, and it started, like with everybody: in his nasal passages. After a week or so, it had gradually moved down to his chest. And not only will it have spread through his chest, but the damage caused by the response to the virus was the reason why he was so badly affected."

Although Dr Tim Fooks could surmise what might be going on with my immune system, other things were much harder to predict. How the illness might respond to certain treatments was very much unknown.

"We all need to remember that there was a collective ignorance, to have that and the inability to be with the person you're concerned about. Understanding that the hospitals were on their knees, wondering what impact that would have. The uncertainty of best treatments, the knowledge that people were dying regularly from this condition, coupled with the disbelief that someone as fit as Laurence might have possibly been affected by this and the real prospect that he might not survive – fifty-fifty was probably a good option – must have made it unbelievably difficult for someone to cope with. You've got to have real depth of character and resource to be able to cope with that sort of level of uncertainty. And very, very few people have to go through it, thankfully." *Dr Tim Fooks*

NHS staff on the front lines in the battle against COVID-19 may not have been experiencing quite the same blackout as I was from within my enforced coma, but they were still manoeuvring somewhat in the dark. As Martine continued to ask questions about the speculated treatments happening in the wider world, it prompted the doctors to suggest she might sign me up to research trials. In the case of COVID-19, research trials were being concocted on the hoof.[14] Obviously, on the basis of a huge amount of knowledge but they were trying all sorts and often with bad side effects like allergic reactions (a bad rash in my case). Also, my own internal immune system went into hyperdrive

---

14 "Maybe clarify that worldwide drugs were used on the hoof, but in the NHS / NIHR, I would say very careful consideration was given to investigating drugs that had a plausible mechanism of action. The only way to scientifically test whether this then translates into a benefit, on average to a person, is to perform a randomised controlled trial, on a suitable number of people. Although performing studies during COVID was challenging, in some ways it was very easy, as so many people had a similar problem. Thus if enough people were recruited, you could definitively say, with a high degree of confidence that X drug works or Y drug does not." *Dr Luke Hodgson*

and was actually attacking me so severely I experienced renal failure and organ shutdowns. The decision was not a small one and ultimately this decision came down to Martine. I was going to be no help.

Tim and Martine discussed the dilemma during one of their phone calls. With his insider knowledge, Tim was able to explain how medical trials worked. This was particularly important in understanding how they were designed in such a way that the data could be interpreted as quickly as possible. Of course, the trials came with challenges. In an ideal world everybody would be allocated the very best treatment for them but when so little is known it is hard to say what that treatment actually is.

"Ultimately all these trials have to be done on the basis of controls and comparing the controls to those that are having the treatment ... A particular thing might work. It might be unsuccessful. It might actually harm someone." *Dr Tim Fooks*

Tim helped Martine understand what was being offered and provided an explanation. "The top and bottom of it is that the nature of the condition and the severity of it meant controlled trials had to be done. It was a difficult decision. First of all, do you risk not participating or do you risk participating? Those are different things. And I think Martine made a good decision."

He added, "From my memory, I don't think Martine ever stopped being rational."

Martine responded, "I did my own research. In France, they were using their own drugs for COVID-19. I asked the experts if they had tried it but I didn't really know what else to ask. I wasn't watching TV, it was all about people dying from COVID-19. It was too much to take in. I asked my sister to keep me in the loop, let me know if there was anything I should be aware of. She told me about the French doctors and their treatments.

When I spoke to the ICU team, I asked them about it. I mentioned my sister had suggested it and I felt embarrassed. I didn't want to tell them how to do their jobs, but I was so desperate. To my surprise, their reaction was different to what I expected. They called me back and asked if I'd be interested in putting Loz into a drug research trial. It was 1st April 2020. I wasn't in an April Fools mood. I told them, yes. I wanted to try anything. Do anything to save him.

I had to make a decision about the drug trial. They wanted to give him a respiratory drug derived from horses, which I later found out about from Dr. Tim. They gave me half an hour to make up my mind. In that short time, I rang Dr. Tim and we talked it over. They had tried it on SARS patients and most of them had died. That didn't help ease my mind at all. Should I or shouldn't I put Loz on the trial? He couldn't make the decision for me. It was all on me. I was lost, drowning in uncertainty, not knowing if this would save him or if it would make things worse. The ICU team called me back after the half hour. There were rules. We had to be flexible. They recorded me authorising it. That same day, Chris Whitty authorised it too. And then the call ended.

The next day, I found out the decision had been made: I had authorised the research trial. They told me he wouldn't be receiving any treatment. One of the research drugs was in tablet form, but they couldn't give him that, as it was a randomised trial [15]from Oxford University. The other two

---

15 "Randomisation: see this explainer from cancer uk https://www.cancerresearchuk.org/about-cancer/find-a-clinical-trial/what-are-clinical-trials/randomised-trials." Dr Luke Hodgson

options were random as well and they didn't know which one he would get.

The ICU sent all the details to Oxford, and they came back with the news of which drug trial he would be placed on. But then they told me it would be *on usual care*, meaning he would receive a placebo. The trial was a test to compare the effects of the three drugs and the placebo. So, after everything: the stress, the worry, the waiting, I got the news that, despite all the research, he still wasn't going to receive any new drug. I was utterly shattered. I felt so disappointed. After all that uncertainty, all the decisions, all the stress about these drugs, I found out he wasn't going to get anything." *Martine Penn*

"Importantly at the time, a lot of experts, based on retrospective observational data, thought that steroids could be *harmful* in the treatment of a virus. Indeed, a lot of consultants did not want to take part in the study testing steroids as they believed, based on previous evidence and their expertise, that steroids could do more harm than good." *Dr Luke Hodgson*

Chapter 5
Guarded in Groundhog Day

After a couple of days my status had not improved. I was, as Dr Hodgson put it, *stably bad*. The medical notes say Martine was being told my condition was guarded. Apparently, that is doctor speak for *touch and go*. Luke Hodgson referred to it as like Groundhog Day. Almost a week went by with very little change. Sometimes I got marginally better. Sometimes marginally worse.

It was on a worse swing when my family were told to get my affairs in order. Martine and Mischa listened to the doctor on speaker phone as he said they didn't think I was going to make it. My family should prepare themselves to say their goodbyes.

"I think my mum, as much as she says she's OK with it, it's obviously one of the most traumatic things for her. Bless her and I think she's found her own way of dealing with it, but do you ever deal with it?

They were basically telling us each day about how he was getting on, his progress, how he's reacting to the medicines and the stuff that they're doing like flipping him on to his back and then his front to try and get more oxygen in his lungs.

On day one, they were thinking it looks pretty consistent and then by day four or five they were thinking he was going south. They didn't think he was going to make it after day five and they were telling us that by saying they're going to start making preparations. They didn't outright say he's going to die. They said it in a more tactful way: "We don't know if he's going to make it so we're preparing." Well, they've obviously noticed trends in other patients and thought, Laurence is doing the same thing." *Mischa Penn*

If there was ever any doubt, it was now quite clear to everyone: I was critically ill. Except maybe me, as I shifted between darkness and dreams. Very many of my dreams involved Martine. Under non-pandemic circumstances, she would have been around my bedside so that might have been more understandable. The bond I felt with her must have been so strong to keep bringing her into my mind time and time again. Her presence was the pin-prick of light. The hope in the dark.

In one dream, she was running her own nursing business. Nurses surrounded her. It was a massive business. I remember seeing the premises, the people working for her – watching her being super successful. Only then, she took on the persona of an Asian lady. Maybe that was when in *real life* a nurse came to sit with me? I remember trying to say to Martine, "Why are you pretending to be an Asian lady? People are going to rumble you. They're going to know it's you. Why don't you stop? Why are you speaking like that?"

In the *real world*, ever competent Martine was determined to keep trying. She asked if it was possible to transfuse antibodies from the family into me. They all wanted to give blood. To me, that would have sounded quite a good idea. It could give me a boost in beating this thing, couldn't it? But there were lots of studies happening and this wasn't one the hospital was currently doing. Still, the doctors could see how my family were thinking about every possible way they might help.

On the evening of 3rd April, senior consultant Dr Luke

Hodgson was doing the ward round when he noticed that I wasn't looking so good. I had got significantly worse and of course things weren't exactly looking peachy before. Thankfully, there was one practice that had proved successful in Northern Italy, where the hospitals had been overwhelmed with COVID-19 patients.

"We talk about fractions of oxygen that have been delivered by the ventilator. Laurence had gone from about forty-five per cent or 0.45 O_2 to suddenly needing about ninety per cent. Oxygen at high levels is toxic. He was on a very high amount of support, so at that point we did this proning, which is shown to likely improve outcomes because it alters the way the gas exchange occurs with the lungs." *Dr Luke Hodgson*

Proning was something that had come out of previous studies into acute respiratory distress syndrome (ARDS). Some medical professionals had reported it was proving effective in fighting COVID-19 but it was not without its risks.

"You end up putting a person into a position where it potentially could be harmful, particularly if you have a very busy intensive care unit. It can be associated with pressure sores and if the tube dislodges from your mouth when you're on a huge amount of oxygen, that can be catastrophic." *Dr Luke Hodgson*

Proning involves turning you in your bed from lying on your back to your front and then a number of hours later, they turn you from your front, to your back. When they prone you, they have to paralyse you, because even though you are in a coma, your nerves might cause you to move or involuntarily jerk.

Of course, when you are in the state I was, hooked up to

multiple machines, it is even more tricky. There were lines going into my neck, main lining the sedative drug that was keeping me under. You can't mess with that. I needed to stay sedated. Therefore, proning takes a team of people, the decision to do it is not taken lightly.

"It's been shown in good quality studies that people who have severe problems with their lungs, if you prone them for sixteen hours a day for a number of days, they're more likely to survive than those who you don't prone. So, from 3rd of April 2020, we started doing this proning. From teatime until nine o'clock the next morning, he was lying on his belly." *Dr Luke Hodgson*

Physiotherapist, Gemma Stoner, also remembers being involved in my proning, "I remember Laurence was one of the first patients we proned. We put him on his tummy because of his oxygenation being so bad. I think he was actually the first patient that I'd been in the proning team to help turn on to his stomach. That's a task which takes a minimum of five people really, but normally six or seven people, with an airway trained doctor looking after the tube."

She remembers how I was proned for a long time, "You spend at least eighteen hours on your tummy and they move your head from side to side every two to four hours for pressure relief. Obviously, because of gravity, all the fluid finds its way to the head. And I remember he had really, really swollen lips and pressure sores. And that was my first memory of Laurence, him having these really swollen lips and sore nose."

It's not normal to spend eighteen hours on your tummy. The drugs can also affect a person's circulation. Add in all the factors and I had a really swollen face. I probably looked rather shocking. Maybe I could have starred in a B-movie, but only if it was a horror.

Besides it being a rather uncomfortable process for my body, apparently, I generally responded well to being proned. The level of oxygen I needed came down a bit, so a plan was made to re-prone me the next evening. Still, things weren't looking great. The doctor told Martine that if I continued to deteriorate, I still may not recover.

"Then came the call. The one I never thought I'd get. They told me they didn't expect him to make it through the night. 'You need to be prepared. He might not survive.' Up until then, I'd been updating Yaz, Mischa, family and friends, sharing every bit of news, doing what I'd promised. But this time, I couldn't do it. I didn't have the strength. The thought of telling anyone what was happening, of putting those words out into the world, it felt like too much. I couldn't bring myself to say it. So, I just ... lay down. Escaped for a moment. Shut my eyes and tried to process, even though I couldn't make sense of any of it. My body, my mind, everything was frozen. I had no idea how to keep going. But I had no choice but to try." *Martine Penn*

I can't imagine what that was like for her to hear. She must have been desperate, clutching at any straws. She asked about the studies. As the recovery study I had been put into had only just started, it could be months before anything came back regarding results. Did I have that long? Did I have weeks? Days? Hours?

Chapter 6
A change of scene

My experiences on HDU suggested it was busy but I only had a very small part of that story. More and more patients needed urgent attention. Normally in ICU it is one-to-one nursing care. That means throughout twenty-four hours of the day there is a nurse at the bedside all the time. As the pandemic raged on, it was becoming more like one-to-two beds or sometimes even one-to-three. Nurses found themselves looking after multiple patients. The unit pulled as many previous ICU workers as they could back to the wards. They also drafted in help from nursing staff who normally worked in different areas.

"Like with any sort of situation, like in a disaster, all sorts of people were wanting to be helpful, weren't they? Whether it was doctors coming from different specialities, there were all sorts of help being suggested. All the rotas had to change. Consultants, who would normally work in the day and then let the team of registrars take over, were doing night shifts. As consultants did night shifts, as well as the juniors, there were lots of doctors around all of the time." *Dr Luke Hodgson*

Also watching intently, what was going on for me, as well as watching patients like me, was Sam Morfee. She had worked as a Theatre Recovery nurse before the pandemic hit but she had moved to help in HDU and ICU as the first wave of COVID-19 hit. To start with, Sam looked after the HDU patients who were on the CPAP masks and hoods. Remember the space helmet I threw up in? That was a CPAP hood.

As the pandemic progressed Sam found herself taking care of ICU patients when other members of staff went on breaks. This meant patients on ventilators, as I currently was. Working in a completely different area had its challenges. There were lots of criteria she had to check and sometimes she felt out of her depth.

"I think it was a case of: this is what we've got to do. We've got to just try and help these patients, and if we don't know what we're doing, we just ask for help. If we didn't know and the other staff members didn't know, then we all just helped each other. It was a case of all hands-on-deck, let's go." *Sam Morfee*

Theatre Recovery – the area Sam was from – is post-surgery care. People coming round from operations. In pre-coronavirus times, Sam would give them pain relief, make sure they were comfortable and then move them back to the ward. However, during the pandemic many surgical procedures had to be cancelled, most particularly routine ones. It meant there were a lot of empty spaces in some wards, like endoscopy. Some of these areas were taken over for other purposes. Patients free of the virus ended up being looked after in what was normally the theatre recovery area. Even though COVID-19 gave the impression that it was the only thing going on, people were still having heart attacks and other health emergencies.

Those with the virus had to be isolated. Sam told me there were red areas denoted round the hospital. There was a red lift if patients with COVID-19 needed to be moved and there was a green lift for those who were not knowingly infected. For NHS staff working on the hospital wards, a great deal had changed in the conditions they were working under and it was particularly crucially that those working with COVID-19 patients were not spreading the virus or coming into contact with it themselves in a way that could potentially be very harmful to them. Sam told me about the PPE they had to wear for many hours at a time.

"It was a full-on gown, down to the floor. I always double gloved. You put one pair of gloves on with your gown and then you put another one on, so if you needed to take a pair of gloves off, if they got dirty [for example], you'd still have cover on your hands." *Sam Morfee*

ICU staff also wore a net over their hair like they would in theatre. There was a visor and then also a mask. For Sam this came with a couple of extra difficulties. She had to remove her glasses to get a full seal round the mask. She also has a hearing impairment and reads lips, so that was impossible with everyone masked up.

"I wear hearing aids, so it was a case of having to put the net over my ears, but without putting the bands over the back of the hearing aids, where there's the microphone. It was a case of just trial and error to start with as to how [to do it], as to which elastic goes where to make sure I can still hear. I was trying to listen to what people were saying, so I was tending to be quite close up. When the doctors did their rounds, sometimes I'd have to say, 'Can you just slow down to repeat that again, so I can jot it down in the notes?' So, yeah, it was tricky." *Sam Morfee*

Nurses wore masks and full PPE for at least three hours, until having a break. Marks appeared on their faces and their skin was affected. Some people broke out in spots.[16]

Gloves protected their hands but they still got a bit sweaty and the need for frequent washing after and in between left

---

16 photo from https://nurseslabs.com/8-tips-to-avoid-skin-damage-while-wearing-ppe/

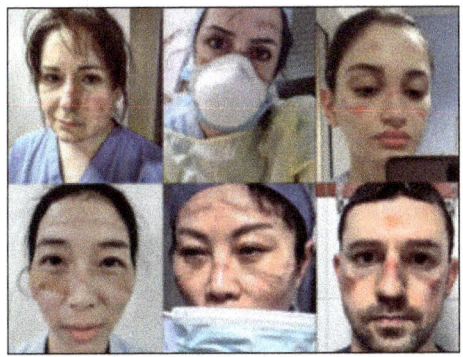

Figure 4 <u>nurseslabs.com</u>

hands dry and sore. When it was hot on the ward, which it was that summer, the many layers made things even more uncomfortable. "So, we had the air conditioning units in the ICU because that was just a warm area. You're literally just wearing underwear underneath, then you've got your scrubs, then your [PPE] on the top." *Sam Morfee*

When the ward staff came out of the isolated area for a break it would be the reverse. "It would be gloves and gown off. Keep your mask on until you're outside. On the other side of the door, there's another bin and a sink. Without touching the main bit [of PPE], take it off, drop it in the bin, go and wash your hands and then breathe and then go and have your breaks." *Sam Morfee*

Breaks would give the staff a chance to refuel. It would also give them an opportunity to attempt to rehydrate. For the three hours they were on the ward they wouldn't be able to drink.

"Normally I would drink throughout the day. I'd take a sealed bottle, and then I'd put it on the side, and I'd drink it during the day. But it's also a case of not over-drinking on your break, because otherwise you need to take everything off to go and have a wee. It's a case of wanting to drink enough so you don't get a headache because obviously it's quite warm, but you don't want to overdrink because you don't want to say in an hour, 'I'm really sorry, I need a wee.'" *Sam Morfee*

I asked Sam how she coped with all this.

"You just think, well, I've just got to get through this till I go for a break. I preferred a later break so at least I could have a sleep." *Sam Morfee*

Sam worked nights, which meant she finished her shift at 8am. It meant she could go home, shower and change in time to drop her son at school.

"I've got quite a high fence up round my garden so I wasn't scaring the neighbours. I'd come home from work and I'd strip off on the doorstep and it would be two or three steps into the house and put everything in the washing machine. My towel would be in the bathroom ready and I'd go through and have a full shower. Then after that, I could give my son a hug before I took him to school. It was a case of we're just being so careful to make sure that we weren't going to infect our families because what we saw in ICU was horrible in some cases." *Sam Morfee*

Cases like me, wired up and confined to bed number one. I continued on, for now, in my enforced coma, with a really swollen face, no doubt looking extremely worse for wear. Sam was watching me and wondering why it was I was lying here in this bed struggling for my life.

"Some cases happened so quickly that it was a shock. You're not thinking that you're going to have so many patients dying in a day. You're thinking, but they were fine when they were sat up talking to me two days ago. Well, how come they're already on a ventilator? What's happened? It was trying to understand why … this is how it's hitting, this is what it is doing and how it's affecting everybody in different ways. Every case was different. And it was thinking, well, is it patients that have got these comorbidities? Or is it ... ?" *Sam Morfee*

About three months prior to the pandemic hitting Worthing Hospital, Sam volunteered to do a COVID-19 course, so she was a little bit more aware as to what was happening and how it was going to affect patients.

"We were planning on having a few extra meetups and going through scenario roles, but the scenario roles actually became real-life roles." *Sam Morfee*

Having taken the course was very useful in practice but it also fed into Sam's curiosity. The COVID-19 course was shocking; it was also a challenging illness to make sense of.

Because she worked nights, this made it a bit easier for Sam to shadow somebody and learn what was going on. During the day, there were physios coming to see patients. By doing the nights, she found she was more able to focus on what the numbers were and understand what they meant. "You'd do a blood gas test and you'd be like, well, are they getting any better? Well, it's a fraction better, but they're up and down. And you could say that they're on the mend and then all of a sudden, the next [day] something else happens. And it's quite touch and go for a lot of patients. It was never a case of we could say, right, anyone over the age of sixty or over the age of forty would be more affected. We got quite a few young ones in as well, so it was all on everybody, really." *Sam Morfee*

I was normally fit and well, why was I so affected?

Sam was asking the questions. What was the criterion for being struck down forcibly by COVID-19? It was a question I too, even in my enforced coma would have really liked an answer to, especially if that answer came complete with an instruction manual on how to get me well again and back home.

Drawing conclusions was hard. It was still early days from a pandemic perspective. It was the first week of April 2020. The population of Britain was confined to their homes, with most shops shut. One hour of exercise outside was all the vast majority of the population were legally allocated.

"I actually didn't mind being out because I had the freedom to go and have a walk along the beach after my shift with a couple of friends I'd worked with. Being in full PPE all the time you're protected. Well, you think … you hope you're a hundred per cent protected, so while walking on the beach in the fresh air any bugs or anything had blown away. The nicest thing was, because I worked with quite a few colleagues who were friends as well, we could give each other a hug with our full PPE on and it was just amazing." *Sam Morfee*

Sam's son still went to school as she was a key worker. It meant that Sam was spared the trials of home-schooling. After she had dropped her son off, she would get in some deep sleep. She would wake up again at three o'clock. Her partner was working from home as he is a sales director for an IT company, so one of them would pick up her son from school and then the family would have dinner together. After dinner, Sam would go to work. She worked two or three nights a week this way.

"It was the little things that actually I didn't mind. I think that's what helped me mentally get through it. It was an experience that was scary. It was an experience that really pushed your boundaries emotionally, mentally and physically, because you don't know what … " *Sam Morfee*

Chapter 7
Critical

Being in a coma for a long time has its risks. I had been ventilated now for ten days and although I had plateaued somewhat since my freefall on day five, I was by no means safe. The nursing staff were working hard, using suction to keep my chest clear of secretions, or as I might have called it *gunk*, and to shift my position to avoid me developing sores. The physios regularly moved my arms and legs, stretching them out to prevent stiffness.

Unfortunately, I had still managed to get a pretty nasty rash and my lips were cracked, despite the best attempts by the ICU nurses to apply Vaseline. Bodies aren't designed for long term sedation. Martine was getting worried. I should say *more* worried. Of course, she was worried about lots of things and rightly so; I was lying in bed number one fighting for my very existence.

My family had been informed that my condition had steadied out a bit. However, they were also told not to get their hopes up just yet.

"You're blank, but you're also feeling everything at the same time, so you think, I'm not going to let myself feel an emotion until I know that he is gone or that he is not. You're in a period of thinking, keep your head level because you don't want to let everything flood in just yet. Do you celebrate too soon? Do you not? Mum and I agreed we're not going to say a word about this. We're not going to celebrate too soon and think that he's coming home tomorrow because obviously we know he's not." *Mischa Penn*

Martine asked the doctors when I might be able to be brought round but was told I was still in a critical condition.

"The protracted nature of COVID-19 was very different to a lot of illnesses on intensive care. Usually, you might have somebody on a ventilator for anywhere between a day to a week or so, whereas with COVID-19 it was much more. You were often stuck there for around a couple of weeks and it was a matter of paying attention to the fine details to try and keep the patient stable and not associated with any [iatrogenic] harms." *Dr Luke Hodgson*

Dr Hodgson explained to me how the longer a person is in intensive care, the more likely iatrogenic harms could occur. These are harms associated with being in hospital. Bugs can get in the system from the lines into veins or those associated with the breathing machine itself – the one currently keeping me alive – pretty important stuff. With me being flat out on the bed, the risk of pressure sores where infections might occur is a concern. The team have to keep all the plates spinning. The battle for my life was not about beating just COVID-19 itself but all the chaos it had created [17].

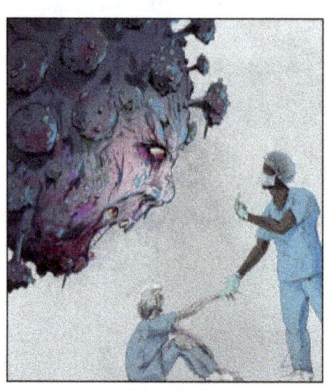

Figure 5
https://www.instagram.com/mjhiblenart/

The team had to explain to Martine that I wasn't ready to be weaned off the ventilator. The ventilator was still doing all

---

17 Not all heroes wear capes, MJ Hiblen Art, illustrator: https://www.instagram.com/mjhiblenart/?hl=en

the work for my lungs and it would have to stay this way for now. Although they did say that at some point I would need a tracheostomy. That means they make a hole in my airway so the tube can go straight to my lungs. A tube in the mouth can be very irritable. They're telling me! A tracheostomy can mean someone is able to be on less sedative agents so I might be more awake and even interact.

This all sounded promising, or it would have done to me if I could have heard it. Unfortunately, I didn't get the memo and on 11th April I got a bit worse. My condition was still very much touch and go. Did I want to go? I did not. I wanted to get out of the hospital and go home. I wanted to see my family. Even in my dreams I was trying to get away, to get from wherever I was to somewhere else I would rather be. I have recollections of a dream on a large boat with many friends and family, I was aware of a chugging diesel motor sound and some lurching movement. In my mind a saw a pier where I could disembark and could sense the boat slowing. I wanted to hustle through all the people, to jump off the boat back to freedom! But no, instead, feelings of huge disappointment as no burst of energy appeared, just a huge sense of not moving, not getting the message from brain to limbs to move.

Martine recalls, "So, after the call with the ICU – gentle voices, calm and kind voices that held the weight of terrible truths – I put the iPad down. I couldn't look at it anymore. I couldn't hold the shape of their words in my head without it spilling over. I went to see my horses.

Why? Instinct. Long before I had language for despair, I had a way of receiving protection, a quiet understanding and holding space that didn't ask questions. As a child, when storms brewed, I slipped out to the stables. I knew how to disappear. That wasn't bravery, it was survival.

Now, older, supposedly grown, I still obey that old choreography. When the world groans too loudly at the seams, I escape to the sanctuary of my horses." *Martine Penn*

*

I had been in the coma two weeks now. Was I bored? Probably.

One dream: I was in an aeroplane going to Baltimore. I don't know why I was going to Baltimore. Never before had I *been* to Baltimore, for Christ's sake. And I was stressing because I didn't have a passport. People I knew on the plane were drinking whiskey and there was a bit of a party atmosphere. And I am thinking, I shouldn't be on this bloody plane. I need to be off this plane. "When we land, you guys can all *f*** off* I'm flying back. I've got to get home." And that is just ridiculous. Because normally, I would be enjoying the party and going, yeah, get me into that whiskey.

In every single dream I had this overriding sense that I had to be somewhere else. I was always trying to get away from where I was. Often, I had travelled somewhere and had to get back. Dr Hodgson says travel is quite common as part of the delirium experienced by patients on ICU. The beds make miniscule movements to keep blood flowing round the body and these sensations lead to dreams of journeys in boats and on trains.

"Quite often people think they've been captured on a vessel and they've been out at sea for a long time. We have quite a large contingent of healthcare workers at the hospital, so sometimes when people are in a particular room and they can only see the heads of people walking round, they think they've been kidnapped. All sorts of strange situations have built up in a person's mind, even a year later they think [the experience] they've gone through is very real." *Dr Luke Hodgson*

I was often being taken against my will somewhere, but in my stubbornness, I was always trying to get back ... back to Martine. That goal was creating a great resistance within me. It was my mission to get home. I had many dreams where I felt I was being held hostage, or against my will. A number of times it was my daughters who showed up to save the day. Martine had provided the hospital with some photos. One that was stuck at the end of the bed was of me and my two daughters at a rugby game in Twickenham. It is a brilliant photograph because we are all smiling really cheesily. It was like my daughters had jumped out of that photo and into my dreams to save the day.

In one of these dreams, I had been whisked off to a hotel in some hot sunny place. I was in a wheelchair and I didn't want to be there. Everyone was trying to rip me off or take me somewhere I didn't want to go. My youngest daughter used to train a lot with me in jiu-jitsu and she has got her own black belt. In the dream, I remember her beating people up, getting rid of them for me and actually wheeling me out of the hotel. These dreams were vivid and the cocktail of drugs I was on were responsible for many of them.

"Recurrently, when we see people in the ICU follow-up clinic, or when they talk about their experiences in the patient and relative support groups, they often refer to being kidnapped or they make up this story about being in some strange place and wanting to escape. The mind produces or tries to make sense of a situation that's very odd to them, but to them the scenario they build is very real." *Dr Luke Hodgson*

Both in their early twenties, in reality my daughters were

fighting my corner in different ways. When the pandemic started, Yazzy, my eldest, was isolated away from home. She was working on a high-end farm so had a special pass to look after the animals but with no contact with people. While Mischa, my other daughter had been working in London when her work got shut down. Now at home with Martine they were each other's rocks. Mischa was good at dealing with the many people ringing the house.

In one bizarre dream, I woke up in a super space age hospital. A doctor appeared in front of me. His mask slid up electronically. When he talked to me it turned out he was a very cool guy with a soothing voice. It then felt like I was in a nightclub at the same time. It was like a cross between a hospital, a nightclub and a cinema and there I was with this real funky dude doctor. He was sliding in and out of the room with this amazing visor system and high-tech chair.

The next thing I know, I'm on an aeroplane flying off to some place in America. I can hear this weird noise. It is like a motorboat race and again, I realise I am in a bed somewhere I shouldn't be. I remember shouting for my daughter Mischa, because I saw her walk past the room I was in.

I was really shouting so loud, "Come back and get me."

She looked back, "Yeah, in a minute ..."

"Come and get me now, please!"

And then that dream fizzled out and I remember looking down and seeing my chest covered in sweat. Was that real?

*

On 11th April I was proned again, which is a sign I wasn't doing well. That is a gentle way of saying there were still serious issues and my life was by no means secure. When I was proned again two days later, Martine was told I was *static* ... statically bad. She asked if I could have the radio on. She knows how much I enjoy drumming. Perhaps some music could help.

Proned again on the 15th. Ugh.

If the infectious disease I was skirmishing with had been better known the doctors would have been able to offer Martine some more information. As it was, my prognosis was so difficult to predict. Martine was still taking it on herself to read all the information she could get from the media and from talking to our friend Dr Tim. She asked the team about a new anti-inflammatory drug being used in America but that wasn't something being used on this side of the pond. In America there is a completely different system. Drugs tend to get licenses more quickly. It is a different approach.

Although initial studies for the anti-inflammatory drug had hinted at the benefits, when it was more rigorously tested by the WHO it was found not to be beneficial.

"People are clutching at things: why aren't we giving out these things? But actually, you have to hold firm to try and be, not just scientific, but understand that there are harms associated with things. Obviously, sometimes we end up giving things as last-ditch attempts, but you always have to be cognisant of actually just adding in an extra thing. You might be doing more harm than not doing it, which is probably quite tricky to put across to people." *Dr Luke Hodgson*

Experimenting with treatments was more complicated than we might have hoped. Things from bed number one were looking pretty bleak with no known cures on the horizon. Hope sure seemed in short supply. However, unbeknownst to me, as I lay surrounded by the ICU team, another fight for my life had already begun a crow's flight away, in a house behind a house, at a wobble in the road.

Chapter 8
Research trials and tribulations

Redeployed into research nurse roles during COVID-19, Linda Folkes and Heather Fox first met me through a document detailing my health particulars. I am sure it was riveting stuff! As long as the team could consent for them to be included in the research, every patient admitted with COVID-19 had one of these documents and it could be as many as thirty-five pages deep. This paperwork was so involved the research team felt they knew each patient personally.

They didn't just know whether you were a non-smoker but whether you had *ever* smoked. Heather remembers them having to read through the information on every patient so they had a grasp of who they were, what they did, and who they had ever been.

"You got to know the person because you got to know what job they did and whether they had family, because you also had to consent them. We know that most of the department were particularly traumatised by Laurence being one of the first people to have been so acutely unwell…" *Heather Fox*

"…[and] to be so fit and well and so active and you couldn't have asked for anybody to be more so," added *Linda Folkes*.

My rapid descent into illness had shaken the team. Heather recalled looking round, thinking, "Well, if he's got it, who else is going to get it?"

"At the very beginning it was the unknown. We were all scared. *Everybody* was scared. And it was like, if this can happen to Laurence, we haven't got a chance." *Linda Folkes.*

In those early days, it was easy for the research team to jump onto the no-hope train with its crowded corridors but as dark as the tunnel ahead appeared to be, it dawned on them, for many people they *were* the hope.

To be effective the research team had to recruit people on to the study trials. They tried to get patients on board before they became very ill by visiting them before they were admitted to ICU but like me, the deterioration in many cases was fast. This meant many people were then too sick to opt in themselves so the team would need to approach their relatives.

"Normally when you recruit someone for a research study, you see the patient, you see the relative, if they want them to come along, but you discuss it in person. It was really out of our comfort zone to have to pick up the phone and speak to someone you do not know whose relative is so ill and you're asking them, on top of all this: would they mind being part of a research study

The team would have to be sensitive as many people would see Worthing Hospital was phoning and panic. After all, their relative was receiving intensive care. The research nurse calling would have to get in quickly to say there was nothing to worry about but relatives would inevitably ask for an update on their loved one's condition.

'How is he then?' You felt terrible letting them down. So, you said, 'I'm really sorry. I just don't know.'" *Heather Fox*

The research team also couldn't offer any assurances about the trials either, they didn't know what would work or what would not. They remembered how hard it was for relatives to make these decisions on their loved one's behalf, the same decisions Martine had to make for me.

Although the conversations were difficult, the team found, at least at the start, most agreed to their critically ill loved one being signed up to the research studies.

"... Because there was no hope. That was all we had. That was all we could offer, really, at that time. I say the only thing ... obviously, they're being well looked after, but we really came into our own in research. Everybody wanted to know us. It raised the profile of research and people were on board with it because they knew we had something to offer."
Linda Folkes

With no confirmed treatments for COVID-19, the research team were able to offer a glimmer of hope for relatives like Martine. It wasn't an overnight solution but it did offer the chance of some development down the line.

The push to involve relatives early and get patients consented was helped by Senior Consultant Dr Hodgson due to his interest in research. He pushed for everybody to be on board. It was more usual for ICU to be rather a closed unit that didn't interact much with other areas of the hospital but during this time developing the link with the research team would be crucial.

Linda and Heather felt an isolation from the rest of the hospital in the house they worked in offsite: the house on the second wobble in the road as they referred to it and a house behind a house. From there they were remote and their experience of ICU in their research roles had previously been limited – although Heather had worked on ICU previously – but they now found themselves needing to go there to further the COVID-19 fight.

At least in the early days of the pandemic, making the trip to the hospital was often very emotional and sometimes quite terrifying. There were constant changes. The isolation area grew so rapidly, the *red zone* seemingly ever expanding.

Before COVID-19 hit, Linda was working in Dermatology and would visit different hospitals for her skin clinics. Heather had been in Cardiology, so would go straight up to her clinic and see patients one after another, giving injections for cardiac issues and cholesterol. The circumstances with the pandemic led to their redeployment. Just as with other areas of the hospital, needs must. It was all hands on COVID-19 … well, not literally … not without at least a couple of pairs of gloves.

From their offsite office, research nurses Linda Folkes and Heather Fox were now contributing to the management of clinical trials into COVID-19. What a task! They were no longer working in the autonomous way they had in their specialist areas. Both research nurses found themselves in meetings in the mornings trying to catch up with the rapid changes caused by the global pandemic.

This was the first time the team had all been doing the same thing, as opposed to focusing on their niches. It was fast-paced but it still felt like it worked really well, due in no small part to their manager coordinating effectively. The team were encouraged to support each other and had to work closely together. There was no other way to stay informed.

"Everything was changing so fast. I had a colleague who finished work at two, I finished at four, but only worked alternate days, so every single day we were phoning each other, saying, 'Listen, what's changed since you left at two o'clock is so-and-so …,' and then she'd ring me after she finished, saying, 'Right, just to give you the heads-up this has happened,' because it changed so, so quickly." *Heather Fox*

The fast changes were not just affecting Worthing

Hospital and its patients. There was a much larger butterfly effect to the research being conducted. Heather remembers a particular incident that brought home the scale at which the research studies were implementing change.

"Then one Friday in particular, at ten to four – it was just before I was going home – they said, 'Stop the Dexamethasone arm!' or whichever one that one was, and the next morning it was in the press. One of the doctors here had said they'd got a relative in Australia and they'd changed immediately, so it wasn't that we were just changing things here; we were changing things for the whole world." *Heather Fox*

The UK was very quick to get the ball rolling on research after the pandemic hit. Approximately a hundred hospitals nationwide conducted trials, Worthing Hospital being one of them. Thankfully I met the criteria to participate. Linda added that my humble contribution as I lay comatose in bed number one influenced big changes. Without the patients and the relatives that signed them up we wouldn't have made such progress with understanding COVID-19.

There were three different major studies into COVID-19 the team were juggling.

"There was ISARIC, where for every person that came into hospital with COVID-19, whether it was symptomatic or not, we had to fill in this huge document. Then we had a RECOVERY study, which Laurence was involved in. That was where you had to speak to the relative ... Some patients were put on normal treatment, some were on Dexamethasone, some were on something else. And then there was a third study, which was called Genomic, which was looking at genetics. You'd have two people working on the RECOVERY study[18], then you had most of the

---

[18] Spearheaded by Sir Martin Landray & Sir Peter Horby at Oxford.

department – because it was so intense – on the paperwork heavy one. And then, with Genomic, it was one [person] doing it or the RECOVERY team. So, we had a rota and the manager would go through it. Or we'd all come in, sit down, and have a discussion, who was doing what, who was doing the follow-ups, etcetera, etcetera." *Heather Fox*

It is common with research that from being an idea to implementing it can take a long time. Heather talked about a study she was working on being five years of clinical trials and then a further two years of number crunching and report writing. Due to the sheer numbers involved in the research into COVID-19, along with the reallocation of resources, things were getting done much faster.

The anti-inflammatory drug Hydroxychloroquine, famously championed by Donald Trump, was discussed and added to the trials. You remember this was a drug my wife, Martine, had asked the doctors about. However, after a short period of time it was judged to be ineffective. A recent study has suggested that Hydroxychloroquine did more harm than good, increasing chances of death from COVID-19 by as much as eleven per cent.[19] Although, to be fair to Trump it may have been beneficial in the prevention of COVID[20]!

Eliminating what didn't work was an important part of the process. The quicker healthcare professionals could

---

Rapidly set-up & delivered the first effective treatment for COVID –
Dexamethansone (a steroid), estimated to have saved a million lives within 9 months.
It was also very helpful in showing a variety of drugs did not work &
thus you could avoid exposing people to the potential risks of a drug with confidence.

19 https://www.theguardian.com/world/2024/jan/12/hydroxychloroquine-covid-increase-chance-death-trump

20 https://pmc.ncbi.nlm.nih.gov/articles/PMC11392261/

disregard possible treatments, the more resources there were for trialling what might actually work. As people came up with new ideas they were added to the research as appropriate. The different things that were being trialled were referred to as *arms* and patients like me were randomised onto what arm of treatment they received. So many different arms took place that Heather and Linda couldn't remember them all off the top of their heads. They mentioned Hydroxychloroquine, Dexamethasone, and Convalescent Plasma but the University of Oxford's RECOVERY trial also looked into drugs like Aspirin, Azithromycin, Baricitinib, Colchicine, Dimethyl Fumarate, Lopinavir-Ritonavir, Empagliflozin, Regeneron's Monoclonal Antibody Combination and Tocilizumab.[21]

As with any trial, there had to be a control group which would receive usual care. That was the same care that people who weren't on the study received. If you were on the usual care arm, you wouldn't receive the trial of particular treatments or drugs. Martine was very upset to hear that for one of the studies, I was put on the usual care arm. She hoped that if they threw the kitchen sink at this thing something might stick and it would get me home.

---

21 https://www.recoverytrial.net/results

Chapter 9
Hope and help

Although research nurses like Linda Folkes and Heather Fox were not on the wards day-to-day, they were still following the progress of patients.

"We were actually reading the whole big story. We were following people's journeys. You would come in thinking, I hope this is a good day today and we've got some positivity coming our way. And obviously people were dying and that was just really hard for us, like it was for everybody, but when we were seeing progress, it was just so uplifting." *Linda Folkes*

Linda remembers what it was like to read through all the paperwork that accompanied each person's case.

"One of the things that really sticks in my mind is ... before COVID-19 studies we didn't have access to the intensive care notes. It wasn't open for us to read because we didn't need to. And then when we could because we were looking at obviously finding all the data about our patients. It was the way some of the staff wrote ... It was so tender and it was just so, oh honestly, it really broke my heart. The way they wrote it was so personal and it was just like ... " *Linda Folkes*

"Like they were having a personal conversation with them," said *Heather Fox*.

Linda added, "Yeah. Normally with *usual* medical notes, we've all written up our notes and they're very factual, because we have to just write as they are: *factual*. We don't gloss it up and make it a bit fancy or emotional but these were very, very caring."

These intensive care notes read like a diary so while I lay in a coma, ICU staff were writing what are effectively little letters about how I have been doing and what I have been up to for each of their shifts. These considerate, caring and highly empathetic pieces of writing are like little snapshots, insights into what was going on for my body when my mind was not present. The time came when it was more present and the nurses on ICU would read me sections to help me become orientated. These words came to mean a great deal to me. They helped to account for some of the darkness.

Along with all the other paperwork, it was these notes that Linda, Heather and the Research team were reading day after day. It must have been very emotional. Linda elaborated more on some of her feelings around that time:

"With the RECOVERY study, especially after twenty-eight days of being on the study, you had to do a follow-up with the standard questionnaire, but with us you had to trawl through all the information, so you read everything. And I was doing the follow-ups for quite a while – a couple of weeks for every shift and I didn't realise how low I'd got. I didn't realise the impact it had on me and I just thought, I can't be that selfish to be feeling this when staff are looking after these patients on the ward. I actually went home and couldn't understand my feelings. I understand it when you're a nurse and you're there, you feel that way, but not actually nursing someone and taking all that information in, to feel the way I did ...

And it wasn't until I asked someone, 'Can you help me do a couple of these bits of paper?'... And they said, 'I can't do any more today because it's really affecting me.' And I went, Oh, my goodness. I realised. Someone's saying it and

it allowed me to understand my feelings. Once I got home and worked it through and talked about it, I saw it was OK to feel that way, but I didn't know what it was. I didn't allow myself to acknowledge it, I suppose. We're doing paperwork and going to the wards and giving out the study drugs. We're not actually nursing people, which is alien to us in a way. When you're nursing, you're hands on, so to do it – in a way remotely you think, I should have no right to feel this way."
Linda Folkes

Heather explained how she was struggling as well. Although, she had previously worked on ICU, she realised people go to ICU most often because it is part of their theatre plan and they have swelling or something has gone wrong. It may also be a car accident or a heart attack that has put them there, but, "With COVID-19 what was happening was people were walking into A&E saying, 'I'm really short of breath, I don't feel right.' And then forty-eight hours later, they were dead. When they were put on ICU, you were thinking, but they *walked* in."

I was one of those cases. I may have avoided an end for now but for how long could I keep that up? Unbeknownst to me the research team were rooting for me. They hadn't seen my face but they had read all my particulars. They *felt* they knew me. They saw me as young and the epitome of health and fitness.

My case had Linda and Heather reflecting on their own lives and those of their families and friends. We were all around the same age. Heather said, "If it's affected this young, fit chap, and he's in the first wave, this ill, it could be any one of us. It was really worrying. I had an elderly, frail mother at home and I couldn't go and see her. So even though I live next door, I used to have to ring her. I used to do all her medications, make sure it was a couple of weeks ahead and then take it round as best I could. I'd wipe it with disinfectant and leave it outside." *Heather Fox*

Linda also remembered the fear. "At the beginning when we were briefed it was like, 'This is really awful. This is really bad. Obviously, we've never seen it before. And the hospitals in London, they're overwhelmed. Everyone's dying. You're going to die, basically. Anyone who comes in is going to die.' You're thinking ... you've got this conflict: I'm a nurse and I have got to look after patients, but actually, I want to be at home with my family and protect them all." *Linda Folkes*

"You had to really dig deep, didn't you?" Heather added.

"You did, because and I'm sure everybody felt that. It was like thinking, right, OK, we've all got two hours to live ... What are you going to do with those two hours? And you're thinking, actually I'd just rather be at home with my family." *Linda Folkes*

Further to the inner conflicts many NHS staff were facing, being a research nurse during the pandemic came with its own particular challenges. One major one being, everyone had an opinion on what was going on, Linda remembered, and some people were not always too backward at coming forward.

"I did feel personally cross with some people saying, 'Oh, well, it's not as bad as they're making out.' You're thinking, if only you could see these people lying here, you would not say that. But also, when I went home, I didn't say, 'Oh there's Laurence in bed [one]; he's doing ...' because I still had that professionalism so you couldn't really put over how terrible it was." *Linda Folkes*

It was frustrating for the staff to listen to the conspiracy theories. Did anyone really think, that from the cleaners, all the way through to the consultants, to the administrators, they were fabricating a pandemic? Both Heather and Linda found themselves on the receiving end of seemingly endless questions about the state of things at the hospital. Linda expanded, "I remember a couple of times walking home and as I'm walking up the road – I mean, we've got a really nice little community in my little street – neighbours coming out, sort of like, 'What's it like on the ward? How many have you got?' And they'd want a briefing. They'd ask, 'Is it as bad as they're saying?' [I'd respond] Yeah, it is bad. [they'd reply something like] 'Have the numbers gone up? Have the numbers gone down?' You're thinking, I don't want to overdramatise it and put fear into people. And I'm just saying, Yeah, and it is what they're saying. It is exactly what they're saying.

I thought, whatever media you choose to look at that's where you're going to get it from, because that's where you're going to stay in. And I'd come home and I'd shut the door and I'd think, [ugh sigh] don't ask me for a briefing. And friends would say, 'Oh, you're in research, so, you know. So, what's the lowdown on all this, then? What do they think about this drug? What do they think about that? Why don't they try this?' And all the suggestions that have come my way. 'Why don't you ask them to try this?' I said, I'm helping to collect the data; I'm not doing the research."
Linda Folkes

Heather added, "They kept going on about Trump's drugs, didn't they? So many people saying, 'Well, why don't they try that?' Anyway, they did try it in the end."

"They did, but it was all sorts of things. And then we'd have a lot of people saying, 'Well, it's all to do with vitamin

D deficiency, so you've got to make sure you take extra vitamin D. You've got to do this. You've got to do that.' Whatever came up in the news, everybody would ring me, saying, 'Have you tried it? You need to protect yourself. You need to get this,' And I'm thinking, oh, my goodness me, I'll be Holland and Barrett if I carry on like this.

And when people were saying it only affects these types of people, and you think, No, you're only feeding into what you want to know, and what suits you, and what makes you feel comfortable. That's where you're going. You want to feel safe knowing that, actually, this won't happen to me and this is where I am. I'm safe in my safe place. And you have to respect that too. So, you had challenges all around really."
Linda Folkes

Heather and Linda also talked to me about some of the other public reactions at the time. Although they may not have joined in with the *Clap for the NHS* themselves, it meant an awful lot to them both. They also talked about how the gratitude of their friends and family made them emotional. Heather recollects when she cried one day

"I was trying to get shopping for my mum, because she's vulnerable, so she can't go out at all. Even now, she doesn't go shopping. And I was working all these extra shifts. I had to stand in a queue. I've actually got a back injury, so I can't stand for long periods of time. And I was thinking how am I going to do this? And word got round, 'Oh, if you go to Sainsbury's at six o'clock in the morning with your badge, you'll get in first.' And honestly, I said, 'Is this true? Is it? I've got my badge,' and Linda's saying, 'Yes.' And oh, the relief. Honestly, I did shed some tears.

I know they had lots of flowers which were supposed to have been given for Mothering Sunday, but obviously people couldn't get to the shops. They couldn't do that. But the flowers were all there and they actually said, look, take a bunch of flowers on your way out. And I felt really appalled at the fact that some people complained and said, we don't want flowers, we want a pay rise. And I was thinking, this is something that's going to get thrown away and I actually really, really appreciated it and popped them on the fireplace in my vase. So those little things – and then obviously others started joining in as well, with Morrison – and that made such a difference because we were working long hours. It was stressful." *Heather Fox*

Chapter 10
Separation and steroids

All the nurses I spoke to opened up about their heartbreak regarding the isolation of patients. Linda remembered that there were dementia patients who had no one with them and no way of understanding why. They imagined the separation anxiety to be extreme.

"As a nurse, when somebody is dying you do everything to make them comfortable, to include the families, so that it's all as nice as it possibly can be. I dread to think what it must be like for the relatives having to say their goodbyes with an iPad. That really goes against the grain as a nurse." *Heather Fox*

But both research nurses had to agree that an iPad was better than no iPad. At least some relatives got to see their loved ones one last time.

"Thinking with Laurence ... He's got children. He's got a wife. They're at home. They can't just come in and see him. They can't be there to hold his hand." *Linda Folkes*

Martine's separation from me when I was sick was taking its toll but she was committed to trying to further my cause. She spoke to the doctors about whether my private medical insurance might be put to use but they explained it wasn't a matter of money. Like so many health-related issues, private healthcare was of course something that could be linked to class and means but with COVID-19 no one could pay their way out of the ICU. The doctors informed her that I was in the best possible place. Private provision would still be a long way off. A national health service allows for the Boris Johnson's of the world to be treated, along with the Laurence Penn's, and the many people less well off than myself.

Short of being able to contribute financial resources, Martine had signed me up to multiple drug trials, which was an amazing way for the NHS to find out what worked and what could help other people. It fast tracked the efficacy of what they were working on. They find out a lot about you, what you don't react well to, what you respond to and that benefitted a great many people regardless of their financial status.

On the 16th it was explained to Martine that I was going to need a tracheostomy. There was limited evidence at the time to suggest whether this was the right thing to do with COVID-19 patients because the disease was too new. However, whether it was the right thing to do or not it must have seemed worth a shot because on the 18th I had the tracheostomy.

Friends of mine knew the surgeon doing the operation and wrote to him telling him not to f*** this up. Luckily, even under that kind of pressure, he did not and I emerged back on ICU with a hole having been created below my vocal cords to give access to my lungs. The hope was that the procedure would ease the discomfort to my throat from being on the ventilator, allow for the lifting of my sedation and increase my ability to move. It was hoped that it may even help my condition.

After the tracheostomy was completed, and though the procedure had gone OK, the doctors observed there had been a few steps backwards. Dr Hodgson saw me on the evening of the 18th. He has since explained what state I was in then. One of the markers the team have is a marker of inflammation – the CRP level.

"We can just see, for whatever reason, with what was going on in the process with COVID-19, we'd have these very high CRP levels and traditionally you'd see that as a marker of an infection, but actually a lot of it is around inflammation in the body's response to an infection that is an issue. And so, we didn't have good evidence for it at the time but in previous studies of severe lung injury, overall steroids are probably beneficial, so they have been shown … I actually started the steroids on him that evening when he was still pretty static and there was quite a dramatic improvement over time to that. And certainly, that CRP just shot down. Obviously – you could say – was it doing the tracheostomy that was partly helpful as well, but his lung function essentially just started to improve."

I asked Dr Hodgson why he chose to give me the steroids then.

"I think that was sort of partly reflecting how ill Laurence was, that Laurence was still very stuck. He'd been stuck for nearly three weeks at that juncture with ongoing pretty high levels of support on a ventilator. I think that the steroids were quite an important intervention."

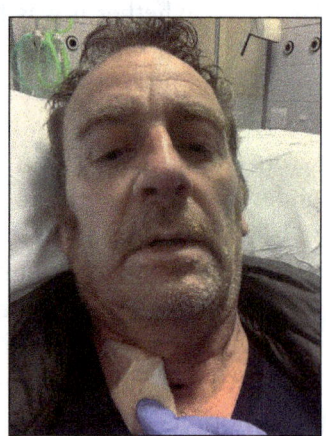

Figure 6

It was by no means a small decision. Dr Tim Fooks explained further:

"It wasn't clear – at the beginning – to determine that steroids were helpful for people with severe respiratory disease, associated with the COVID-19 virus. Steroids are anti-inflammatory. It's a hormone designed to ... produced to enable the body to respond to stress. But one of the impacts of steroids is that they reduce the inflammatory immune response. And so, if the damage was purely due to the virus and people had been given lots of steroids and that had reduced their ability to fight the virus, they would have got worse." *Dr Tim Fooks*.

Chapter 11
Bright lights, prayers and Richard Hammond

In 2006, *Top Gear* presenter Richard Hammond was in a car crash. A really bad one. The Vampire jet-powered dragster car he was driving at the time was going between 288 and 320 miles per hour, according to different reports, when one of the front tyres of the vehicle failed. He was in a coma in Leeds intensive care and claims to have had a vivid dream about the Lake District. In the dream he says he was walking the fells.

"This is a personal story about places, about going places in your mind and I suppose, well, about the power of, well, daydreams ... In my mind I'd been walking these hills here, in the Lake District, overlooking Buttermere. I was having a lovely time strolling along and gradually I got a growing sense ... you know, when you're in trouble? When you're a teenager staying out just that bit too late, you're not definitely in massive trouble yet, but you're in a bit of trouble, and that feeling grew and grew. And I walked up this slope to where I am now, towards this tree, this exact tree and as I got closer and closer to the tree, that sense of 'oh, I really am in trouble. I'm going to be shouted at. I'm going to be in a lot of trouble' grew and grew. Until, eventually, in my dream I turned back. I didn't walk around this tree and carry on. I woke up." *Richard Hammond* from his YouTube video *What*

Really Happened[22].

When he shared his vivid dream with his wife, he learnt that she had been called into the hospital because he wasn't doing very well.

"She was told 'I'm really sorry. Things aren't looking good ... I think you're going to lose him,' and she said, 'Is there anything I can do?' They said 'No, not really,' and she said, 'Can I shout at him?' And they said, 'Yeah, whatever.' And she said, 'No, I mean really, really shout at him?' And she did. And, apparently, she roared and screamed and swore at me, 'Don't you dare die,' and that's when I turned back from this tree in my dream and that's when I woke." *Richard Hammond* from his YouTube video *What Really Happened*

People speculate on whether you can dream when you're in a coma. They wonder whether you can really be aware of anything. Surely, the person in a coma is paralysed? They're out of it. But my experience, like Richard Hammond's, would suggest you are aware. I was aware of voices, of personalities, of energy. I'm convinced they showed up in my dreams.

Also, like Hammond, I had a vivid dream of place. In fields at the back of where I live – where we walk the dogs – there's a large oak tree by a chestnut post and rail fence where the grass grows really long in the summer and you get this lovely sensation of the grass moving, swaying gently back and forth in the gentle summer breeze. In my dream, I saw that as a scene and I remember the dog bouncing along in the long grass. Literally, you must see it for a nanosecond but it feels like it might have been an hour-long movie. I don't know whether that was inspired by the image of my dog on the end of the bed but I do remember thinking I want

---

22 https://www.youtube.com/watch?v=_BYQLDU9xhI

to see that again: I want to run my hands through that lovely long grass and breathe in the sweet hay, grass smell.

Coma dreams are so strong. Maybe it is the morphine; maybe it is the lack of anything else to keep your brain active, but I really felt I had been to the places my mind created for me.

Hammond gets it. He said, "It's true. I mean I didn't really come up and walk around this tree, I was in a coma in Leeds, but my mind did and my mind is who I am. I know that very well having damaged it from a frontal lobe brain injury and spent a long time recovering. And I've taken huge solace from that ever since, because that was my last thought, certainly at the time. And my last thought took me somewhere I love and somewhere I'm happy. And that last thought if I had shut down and stopped would have echoed, as far as I was concerned, for all of eternity. And I've found immense comfort from it ever since." *Richard Hammond from his YouTube video What Really Happened*

Hammond's words speak to my own experiences. My own suggest if you have been ill there is a way out and a way back. For me there was always a pinprick of light, even in those darkest of circumstances. That pinprick of light was always leading back to my wife. We have a very strong relationship and we've been married for thirty years. I've known her for thirty-five. She is hugely important to me, to who I am.

Because of all the precautions around the pandemic, Martine wasn't able to shout at my bedside. I have no doubt if she could have done – if she had thought it would have helped – she would have been there screaming the ward down.

She may not have been there but I just had a sense. What do I mean by that? We have a friend who is a very successful business coach. She coaches senior executives within the NHS, Google and Amex. When you sit down and talk to her you can just tell she has a gift, an immensely positive energy. She can pick up straightaway what the real problems or issues are. Martine had gone to her. She said, "I don't know what more I can do," and this woman said, "We're going to send energy to Laurence."

Well, that was one thing. Another came through my daughter, Mischa who didn't spend lockdown with her partner. She was, as we have heard, back at home with Martine. Mischa's boyfriend is half Italian and his Italian mother is very religious.

My daughter told me, "One night, Josh contacted me and said, 'Right *now*, pray. My mother's family in Italy ... there's a whole church full of people ... they're praying for your dad right now, so just pray.'"

My partner's mum is incredibly spiritual. She's met my dad a couple of times, loves my family, feels very connected to us. She's Italian, so there's a big presence in Rome of Catholics that collect in the church to pray every week and she'd obviously reached out to all of her network to basically say, 'Please, can you pray for my daughter-in-law's father? He's in hospital suffering with COVID-19. Please, can you pray for him?' Many of the churches in a certain area in Rome were all praying for him every single week. I think they did it every day, actually, because they did daily services." *Mischa Penn*

"One day, Mischa and I were sitting quietly in the kitchen when the phone rang. We already knew how badly Italy had been hit by COVID-19, the news reports were grim. It was Mischa's boyfriend's mum calling, her voice steady but filled with urgency. She explained that in Italy, a group healing had been organised, a collective effort to send energy and healing to those suffering from the virus. She told us that we were to sit together, hold hands, and as a group, send Loz healing energy.

We exchanged a look, unsure but desperate. We had reached a point where we would grasp at anything that might offer some hope. So, Mischa and I sat together in the kitchen, holding hands. Our minds torn between doubt and the faintest glimmer of belief. We did our best to follow Sabina's suggestion, trying to channel everything we had: our love, our hope, our longing for him to recover, into that moment. It felt awkward at first, almost surreal, as if we were hoping for something that could never be, but we did it anyway.

In that moment, time seemed to stretch and all we could hold onto was the smallest thread of belief: somehow, in some inexplicable way, this act of sending him energy could make a difference. It was our only option, our last thread of hope. And so, we held on to it with everything we had.

After that call, we couldn't keep it to ourselves. Every person we spoke to about it, we shared what we had done, this small, almost desperate act of sending healing energy. And without hesitation, everyone we told got on board. They said they would do the same, that they would join us in this group healing, sending their love and positive energy to Loz, no matter how small the gesture might seem.

It was a strange comfort to know that others were willing to be a part of this, even if it felt uncertain. It felt like, in the face of all the fear and helplessness, we weren't alone. We had all come together, in our own way, to support him. To hope for his recovery. Each person who joined in was another thread in the tapestry of hope we were trying to weave for him.

The next day, the ICU called. As I spoke with them, I couldn't help but share what we had done. I told them, 'We've been sending him energy healing. I added, half laughing and half in disbelief at myself, 'With the amount of energy healing his family and friends have sent by now, he should be up and running round the ward!' I paused, feeling the weight of it all, and then I said, 'You must think I'm bonkers, but this is the only thing I can do right now, being stuck at home.'

There was a brief silence on the other end, as if they didn't quite know how to respond. I laughed a little, trying to keep the mood light, but inside, I was drowning in frustration. It wasn't much – this act of sending healing – but it was the only thing I could offer, the only thing that felt like it might have some small chance of making a difference." *Martine Penn*

*

I'm not a religious guy. I would have to describe myself as an atheist but that doesn't mean to say I don't believe in something spiritual. I do. I just don't believe it resides in a stone church somewhere. I can't see that. Science doesn't support it, so my atheism to me isn't the lack of belief of a God. It is a belief in a different energy altogether.

What I do know is I felt something. I remember *something*. I remember this feeling of good and being able to sense light, energy, feeling *backed* by something and thinking I am going to be OK. I am going to get out of this.

Of course, I didn't know all this praying in my name was going on but I do remember experiencing this light and this energy. I don't know where that came from. Whether that was the drugs I don't know. I can't explain that. It was very spiritual.

"Yeah, Dad does remember feeling lots of light and presence and in some of his dreams was saying that he felt like someone was there telling him, 'It's all going to be OK,' things like that, which is really, really lovely. Obviously, we were all doing our bit to send him healing and our love. 'We're there, you've got this.'" *Mischa Penn*

If there is a way of transferring energy through care, through support, or through praying, whatever you want to call it, I definitely received some of that. I am well aware. I can just describe it as good energy.

"We've never been religious as a family but when things happen like that and then Dad says, 'Yeah, I felt an overwhelming surge of light.' It makes you think, oh, God, oh, *God*. Do I need to believe in God?" *Mischa Penn*

I think it is affirmation, isn't it? Sometimes praying for something is almost like trying to manifest it. If you think: I really want that to happen, then you have visualised it and some people say the brain knows no different than real and imagined. You are willing it to already have happened. Athletes, businesspeople, sports people, even high functioning Special Forces soldiers will visualise something in detail, whether it be a toboggan run or parachuting into an area. Frame by frame they will visualise it.

I think by visualising it, it gives it reality. You can start to believe in it. It is almost like putting it out into the universe and it will happen. And if it doesn't happen, I'll learn from that and try again. The brain is an incredible piece of kit.

Being in a coma is rather a lonely business consciousness-wise but even when you come round you can feel a lot of detachment. How do you explain what you have been through during so much overwhelming darkness? How would I be able to explain the wanderings of my mind, the energies I felt, the feelings of being pulled this way and that?

It would take a while, but I recently met a chap whom I discovered had been in a horrific accident at work when he was in his early twenties. He was working on a vehicle, with a full tank of fuel, when a spark from a welding device ignited, engulfing him in burning petrol. He was so badly burned he spent a year in hospital, two months of which was in a coma.

He asked me, "Did you see the light or sense the light?"

We were on a post-pandemic sailing trip with mutual friends. Now, this is the only time I had spoken to someone who had also been through a coma since my hospital stay.

"Yes," I said with an intonation in my voice that I hoped conveyed: you too?

He smiled at me and said, "Yeah, I was aware of being drawn towards a light and having an overwhelming feeling: it's not your time; get out of here! And I came round."

Hearing this, something in my brain clicked into place. It had been hard making sense of my own experiences. How can you make sense of an enormous energy, a positivity, a knowing, a light that powers you on to consciousness?

We both laughed at this, at the *knowing*.

Chapter 12
Martine and reality

With the tracheostomy doing its thing, the steroids reducing the inflammation in my lungs and my battle with a bright white light behind me, things started to look just a little bit more promising. A swab was taken and it read negative for COVID-19. The staff didn't take it as a one hundred per cent guarantee but it looked like I had cleared the virus.

There was even talk about weaning me out of the coma. Firstly though, Martine was offered the chance to have a video call with me. How daunting must that have been? Previously, Martine had declined the offer of a video call. I think seeing me lying motionless in bed connected to various machines bleeping away and the sound of the ventilator would have been too much but now she was keen to see me and most particularly before I was awake so she could support me through coming off sedation. The doctors explained that Martine may find seeing me distressing. I would have changed a great deal in the three weeks I had been in the coma.

On 20th April 2020 Martine and Mischa saw me again over a video call. The nurses had sent some photos but here was the live feed.

"It was odd to see someone fully tubed up, lying in a bed, looking lifeless and you're speaking to them, trying to act all happy and say nice things because that's what they tell you to do. 'Oh,' I say, 'Hello, it's Mischa and it's Mum here; we're here.' The whole time I'm thinking, I would never speak to him like this.

It was tough to see it for the first couple of times. I really struggled, as did Mum, but obviously Mum puts on a brave face because she's a very strong woman. You never get used to it, really, do you? But they did all they could to make it a nice experience and tried to get us to have as much FaceTime as possible with Dad and the hospital staff. Sometimes I said, 'Mum, I'll let you do this one because I don't think I can do it.'" *Mischa Penn*

"Mischa and I hugged after the recording, holding each other tightly. She had been crying, but somehow, she managed to pull herself together. We were supporting each other in that moment, both completely overwhelmed by what we had just done. I could feel the weight of everything pressing down on us. Mischa had taken a photo of Loz during the recording and sent it to Yasmine. Later, I found out it had ripped her apart seeing her dad like that—unresponsive, lying in a coma. She had been so strong up until that point, holding it together, but that photo was her reality check and it shattered her.

Mischa and I were trying to console each other, but it felt impossible to find any words of comfort that could ease the pain of what we had just witnessed. We were both lost in the emotional weight of it all." *Martine Penn*

*

Hearing familiar voices, seeing known faces is considered very important to help with mental recovery of people coming out of comas, especially when trying to reduce someone's delirium, so these FaceTime sessions were considered vital. I had been sedated a long time by most standards. Martine was also worrying about my mental health. That is her thing. She is an Equine Assisted Psychotherapist and fully trained in Human Psychology. Her fears were not irrational. How would I react? When they brought me around would I panic? Would my fight or flight mechanism kick in?

Dr Hodgson explained to me how people who are quite delirious can potentially try to pull out the lines that are attached to a massive blood vessel or to a person's tracheostomy. That's potentially catastrophic so the staff try to keep someone in a safe state and sometimes medications are used more in intensive care than in other parts of the hospital.

Being weaned out of a coma is a very disorientating process. As sedation is reduced you slip in and out of consciousness. It is very hard to keep a grasp on what is real. My sense of reality was made all the more shaky by the vivid dreams that flooded into the space between being asleep and awake. I'm not sure now which dreams took place while I was still sedated and which came as I was coming round.

There's one particular really vivid dream I had where it felt like I was in a place that resembled Canary Wharf. I had travelled across the water. I was in a restaurant. One that I felt I shouldn't have been in. It was very swanky and dimly lit, with staff efficiently marching round. I had this dish of food. It was dim sum of some sort. I don't know who I was with. And I remember standing up and leaving the restaurant, going from dimly lit to a much brighter light. I had the sensation of tripping over and face planted on to the ground. I felt really uncomfortable, unable to move … at all! I could see myself in a bird's eye view. I was looking down at myself, sprawled on the ground. Then there was a newspaper article with the headline reading: MAN MISSING FOR THREE WEEKS. UK WIDE HUNT.

I wanted to speak out, "I'm here. I'm fine. I'm all right."

But no sound came out. My frustration was through the roof. I wanted to shout, to scream but not a sound or movement could I make.

The next thing I knew, I was lying on my back looking up and someone wearing a mask and blue clothes was holding my hand. I remember seeing the hospital ceiling. Those hospital ceilings I will never forget. They have got lights all over them and they are gridded. I remember seeing this guy looking at me, against the backdrop of ceiling and saying, "It's OK, Loz, we're looking after you. You're fine; we're looking after you." And I wanted to say something, but I couldn't speak.

I had the overriding sense that I wasn't in this country, I was abroad somewhere, being held against my will in some sort of bizarre experiment. I needed to let my wife know that I was OK and I was going to get home. It was such a vivid dream I could almost paint the details of the guy's face. I wanted to be rude to him, I was raging. "Let me get the f*** out of here."

But I couldn't. I couldn't do anything. I just looked at him as he tried to reassure me, as he held my hand. That sense of not being able to move, not being able to speak was horrible.

*

"One day, I got a call from an ICU nurse named Gemma. She said they were preparing to bring Loz out of his coma and she would be the one sitting with him. The first face he'd see. In normal times, that would've been me or someone close. But these weren't normal times. Full PPE, masks, gloves, everything designed to protect, but also creating such distance.

Gemma was so kind. She explained that patients often come out of comas in a combative state, not because they're angry, but because they're scared and confused. She wanted to help make that moment less frightening, so she asked me to tell her about Loz.

I said, 'You better have a big piece of paper!' Because Loz is full of life and impossible to summarise. She asked if he was retired, I laughed, 'No! He's a sales director at a big company!' Then I told her about his black belt in Brazilian jiu-jitsu (and joked she might want to watch out), his love of cycling, sailing and especially his puppy – which was his birthday present from the year before. That Loz is the gentlest soul, with a brilliant sense of humour.

It meant so much to be asked about him, not as a patient, but as a person. To know Gemma cared enough to bring *him* into that room, not just his medical chart. In all the fear and chaos, that moment felt like a gift. I knew he was in good hands. And even behind the mask and visor, I knew Loz would feel that too." *Martine Penn*

*

On 21st April I opened my eyes properly for the first time that month. To the medical observers present, I appeared settled but they couldn't tell what I was registering. What I made of them I am unable to tell you because I can't remember. Bed number one in ICU was in a place where it got a lot of foot traffic. Dr Hodgson described it as like a *corridor effect*, all sorts of people would have been going back and forth past my bed and this may have had an impact on my dreams.

As I was stirring from my coma, falling in and out of sleep, the environment and the NHS staff around me came to me in my dreams very often. The machines that kept up their rhythmic beeping would sound out through my coma fog. Then there were no-contact bins which banged shut regularly. Bang! Bang! In a dream, that could become a gun shot or something else noisy and abrupt.

One of the doctors in the ICU team must have had a vague resemblance to Alan Partridge, because to me Alan Partridge really was looking after me. He and I were talking about developing a remake of *The Persuaders*. Made in the early 70s, the original was a British television series that starred Tony Curtis and Roger Moore. They played an unlikely duo brought together to right wrongs and protect the innocent.

What was that about? Was it a dream? Was it a real conversation? Was there even a doctor who looked like Steve Coogan or did I watch *I'm Alan Partridge* on TV, fall back into a drug-induced sleep and make it all up? I don't know.

My grasp of reality surrounding people was as dubious as my concept of space. In one dream I went through a door on the hospital ward, one I imagined to be there. On the other side was a passage to the beach. I am sat there with a good friend of ours, Dawn. We were chatting and having gin and tonic. It was really nice and sociable.

And then Dawn said, "I just need to put a line in you."

"Dawn, no, no. I've had enough of that. No more."

And she replied, "No, I need to put one in."

Obviously in the *real world* it was a nurse trying to put something in my arm.

"No, Dawn, f***'s sake. Don't do it." In my dream I felt myself getting angry.

My wife had warned the hospital staff, "Laurence does jiu-jitsu and he knows some pretty good moves."

I know a lot of wrist locks. Very, subtle wrist locks, but with a move like that I could put someone on their back. You wouldn't think it, but your wrist only goes so far. If you put power behind it, the rest of the body wants to follow.

Some people do wake up from comas swinging because

they are so confused about where they are. How much was real and how much was dreaming, I don't know. I can't distinguish between that which happened and that which did not. It all feels real to me because to me, in my mind, it happened.

A constant reality for me in both the dream world, the real world and the space in between was that bloody bed I was in. I would *wake up* and see this same bed I was wired up in again and again. Once I thought I was in a ski area somewhere in the mountains, in a lobby where people were coming and going with skis. And I am there in my bed and I am asking for food. There is a guy saying, "Yeah, I've got some lovely Indian food. We're going to make this lovely Indian bread and you can have some." Ah brilliant, I think.

"Why are we in a ski lodge? Why are we at the top of a mountain?"

Chapter 13
Delirium, delusion and FaceTiming

On the 22nd it was acknowledged by the doctors that I was constipated. They were telling me! I was having lots of dreams about escaping to the sea so I could take a poo in the ocean. Morphine jams you up.

In ICU you are constantly looked after by a team of nurses, anaesthetists, consultants, doctors, respiratory physios and an impressive array of technical medical equipment. They have got you, from the times where I was in and out of consciousness using a trachea to breathe, to: once the team were confident I could breathe for myself, to: being gradually weaned off strong sedation. When the trachea was removed it left a hole in my throat that was then covered with a large skin coloured plaster. At this stage I was still hooked up to drips for fluids, a tube was still going through my nose into my stomach providing liquid foods and a catheter was fitted for peeing. Pooing is another story.

When they bring you out of sedation, you are still blitzed and pretty floppy. In the moments where I was lucid, all sorts of people were coming over to bed number one and air high-fiving me saying, "Well done!" and "You pulled through! You had us worried there."

I looked at these extraordinary people in a state of total bewilderment. I literally still had no clue or genuine understanding what they were talking about. I flitted in and out of consciousness. It was all I seemed to do.

I woke to someone else at my bedside.

"You don't remember me, do you?" said a consultant.

She started to explain that she was with the team proning me. It was true I didn't remember her but in an instant her voice was familiar, soothing, encouraging, but I struggled to say something back. I couldn't. I had no voice. I smiled instead. My lips cracked, as dry and sore as they were. The fog was returning as she smiled and was off. The constant hum, beeping, bashing of bin lids, voices all merged into one noise as I slipped off again into a fitful sleep, fighting reality.

In the very slowly clearing fog, my brain was still thinking I've been out for a couple of days but my lungs and most of my body had taken a complete hammering. I was not able to be up and about. My lungs needed to be *cleared* regularly. From what I could tell, the respiratory physios peeled back the plaster covering the hole where the tracheostomy was and inserted something that created an almighty urge to violently cough which inevitably brought up phlegm that was hanging round in my lungs. In other words, they used a small hoovering device for sucking away all the revolting phlegm. It's a horrible process but necessary, I was assured. This was incredibly tiring and once done I was not much good for anything and fell back into dream riddled sleep.

Mischa remembers how hard it was to talk to me on the video calls once I had awoken. She said it was in some ways much worse than before.

"Oh, God! It was like speaking to someone who, although their eyes are open they're not there. That's what it felt like. They were trying to get him to do a thumbs-up. To show he understands. That just breaks my heart because that's my dad, and all he can do right now is give me a thumbs-up. That was probably the worst part because you know he's in there, but he's also not in there. And the nurses talk to him like, 'Laurence, can you give a thumbs-up, please?' They talk to him like a baby. I found that difficult." *Mischa Penn*

Mischa acknowledged that how the nurses spoke to me felt alien to her at the time but it was all I could manage.

"How could they have known? They were just doing what they thought was right. I know that Dad was none the wiser because he was almost in a state of vegetation, if you will, but he would probably have found that funny, knowing they were speaking to him like that. That was how I had to think about it: it's a funny situation, he is awake, he's alive and they're just trying to make things simple for him." *Mischa Penn*

The nursing staff encouraged my wife and my daughter to speak to me through the regular video calls and say, "How are you doing?" and "You're doing well." I had no idea what they were really talking about. My wife told me then how I was her hero and how much she loved me and was wishing for me to get better every day, so I could come home.

As I became a bit more aware, I was suddenly able to see. Like a faithful old diesel engine my brain chugged into life, "My God, it's my wife!" It was like I had just completed a very small part of a jigsaw puzzle. I knew, there were a ton more pieces to place but it was a start. Nursing staff said I had tears in my eyes. They were saying to me, "You just need to relax and you'll work it out and you're going to get better. You are going to be here with us for a few more days though, because you're not out of the woods yet."

To prove what they were saying was true, later that day they had to sedate me again because I was breathing really fast. One of the nurses found a radio so I could listen to some music to help me relax.

Sitting up in a chair for an hour would wipe me out but

it was all incremental progress. In one of those early video calls when I was still unable to talk because I didn't have a speaking valve installed, they instead gave me access to a whiteboard where they had drawn out the letters of the alphabet. All I had to do was point to a letter and they would write it down. I say all! At this stage, I was still not really with it. I was still thinking: I am in some kind of a dream, being held against my will in some institution. For some stupid reason, I thought we were in Wales. I *knew* my car was in a car park in Wales.

There were three nurses around me and my wife on an iPad watching this and slowly I spelled out: c-a-r k-e-y-s. It took ages to get there because you wouldn't think it but that marker pen, to me, felt like I was trying to lift up an iron bar. Still, I persevered. This was important: car keys.

And they were all laughing and my wife was laughing. And in my head, I thought, what is so bloody funny? They will get my car keys. I'll be able to go and get the car and I'll be able to drive home. And get out of here.

The physios were saying, Laurence you can't walk. I hadn't been out of bed for yonks but I still hadn't totally comprehended what was going on. It just felt like it was a dream. I was going to wake up soon. The hilarious laughter faded as I closed my eyes.

"The doctors called me on FaceTime through Microsoft Teams. By now, I was a bit of a whiz on Teams.

When I answered, Loz was sitting up in bed. He had a tracheotomy in and was struggling to speak. I couldn't hear him – it was distressing for both of us – the trachea wasn't working properly.

The nurses were trying to interpret, and so was I, but the more he tried, the more air was just rushing into his lungs, no words were coming out.

One of the nurses handed him a board with letters and a pen, something they must have used before in situations like this.

He started to spell something. The board said: car.

I was confused. I thought he meant Carr – my sister's married name. I told him they were fine. 'It's OK,' I reassured him.

Then I saw he had written: keys.

I said, "The car is fine." But I could see he was getting more distressed.

I was distraught. He was getting more upset, more exhausted. So, we left it there and ended the call.

I sat in my kitchen, in my thoughts, feeling the call had done more harm than good for him." *Martine Penn*

Amelia Palmer, team leader of the respiratory physios, has a slightly different memory of this exchange, which is to be expected. I was still pretty out of it. She remembers me talking so maybe it was a bit later on.

"Laurence was trying to talk to Martine and the girls on the iPad. We were holding it up for him. But he was trying to say to Martine, 'Get my keys. I need the keys. If you find me the car keys …' He thought he was going to drive his car out of wherever he was trapped. He didn't really understand where he was but he knew that he wanted to get away, which was just very sweet.

It is the kind of thing that we see quite a lot: people wake up and they are very confused. They often feel they are being held against their will in some sort of prison. Often, they can see that it's some sort of *medical* prison, but they don't often think they're in a hospital. They do maybe feel that they've got to fight for their life.

What we see sometimes is people know they don't want us to *know* that *they know* they're being kept prisoner. Therefore, he felt he couldn't let me hear. He was indicating: get me out of here. I need you to get the keys. And Martine was trying to explain to him, 'Don't worry, you just need to focus on getting better.' And he was doing an aside through gritted teeth, 'Get the keys.'

Yeah, it was very funny to look back at that one. I told him that story. Obviously, he doesn't remember. And I think Martine said that he had started to text her some weird messages as well." *Amelia Palmer*

*

I was slowly discovering that I had been in a coma for most of April. I knew that I felt pretty beaten up, weak and I couldn't speak. My throat and mouth felt really sore and dry. I still had a feeding tube up my nose, a catheter and I was hooked up to various monitors bleeping away.

Everything seemed vague apart from the positivity of the NHS staff. They were telling me I was doing great but I tried to lift my arms and they felt super heavy. Literally everything was an effort. Thinking was draining so I would go off to sleep again.

Martine was worried I seemed so tired. The doctors expected it on account of how I was using my own lungs more. They felt the main issue at the moment was my delirium. I was getting agitated intermittently so they started me on temporary anti-psychotic medication to reduce my distress. I was apparently trying to communicate, but I couldn't write clearly. I was obviously muddled.

It was such a very strange environment with no visitors allowed and all the staff wearing masks and full PPE gear but I started to recognise eyes and name badges. You can tell people are smiling by the lines round the outer edges of their eyes. It's a great feeling to sense that people are genuinely pleased with you but also confusing not to know why.

At that point you see how amazing all the nurses are because they take the time to sit down and talk to you. They just tell you what you have been through and that you have done really well. When someone says to you: you have done amazingly, that you're a real fighter, it is somewhat confusing though. I am thinking, I have no idea what you're talking about. They might as well have said, "Welcome to planet Earth, Mr. Zorg." That might have made more sense.

*

Here are some entries from the patient diary:

9th April 2020 Hi Laurence, today you have had a good comfortable day. You still have a tube in your mouth which is connected to a ventilator and is helping you to breathe, your oxygen demand has reduced which is positive. We have turned the sedation off this morning and been watching how you respond. Your lips are swollen from where you have been laying on your front (proned). I have made sure your mouth is clean and not dry. I have put mouth gel inside your mouth and Vaseline on your lips. I have changed your position every couple of hours to make sure you don't get any sores on your body. You are no longer requiring medication to support your blood pressure, which is great. All small steps in the right direction. The physios have seen you twice today and suctioned the secretions on your chest, they are still there and we are managing to suction them off when possible. You have had regular nebulisers today which has helped. It is now 19:00 and we had to restart your sedation because you are not breathing with the ventilator, you are against it.

15th April 2020, 17:40 It's Roni and Letty here, we are the nurses looking after you today. You have had a good day and have been pretty settled. We turned you from your stomach to your back and we have been able to reduce your oxygen a little. You are still sedated and the ventilator is breathing for you but you are making small steps in the right direction, keep going! Roni and Letty, x

*

I have since asked Luke Hodgson about patients coming round in ICU and how they might be affected cognitively.

"We know from lots of big studies of patients on intensive care, if you're ill, at least thirty per cent of people have a delirium. So, your brain functioning is disrupted and that's multifactorial, a mixture of the illness itself making your body very ill, so your mind doesn't work as normal, but then mixed into that your sleep-wake cycle is disrupted and you're on lots of different drugs. Initially, and particularly with COVID-19, when people are very unwell, to help with work with the ventilator and also to sort of manage the patient when they're in what's called a prone position, they would be on quite strong sedatives, which are actually also associated with delirium and sometimes pain as well. It's a mixture of unfamiliar surroundings and all those things. Delirium is very common. And I think COVID-19, the virus itself, was probably associated with an increased level of delirium." *Dr Luke Hodgson*

I was interested in asking Luke more about how staff helped in the process of weaning and supporting patients like me who were experiencing delirium. He said a lot of it was about reassurance and reorientation, so telling patients that they are in hospital, that it is this day, this time, this is what we are going to do and then sort of repeating that over the course of the day. They also try to keep similar nurses

Delirium, delusion and FaceTiming

looking after a person for familiarity.

"We don't try and force people to stop believing in whatever but try to work with them to understand what it is. We know in cases of delirium, about eighty per cent of them have what is called a hypoactive delirium where the person tends to be very quiet and is sort of looking at people a little bit suspiciously. They've gone inside their head, where there's a lot going on, while being very confused. But outwardly you might not notice that person is very confused without specifically questioning them." *Dr Luke Hodgson*

The ICU team screen for this kind of delirium regularly because a patient might not be presenting as confused. They might even be following basic instructions. I was. Although I was also appearing fidgety and frustrated in between bouts of sleep.

I had a dream my younger sister was marrying into a huge family and I was trying to stop it because I thought it was a scam and they were just after my dad's money, even though in reality he didn't have any! One of them gave me a gift of a pair of socks. When I woke up from that dream, I was wearing the socks. I was *actually* wearing the socks. They were hospital-issue socks with rubbery soles to make falling over less likely. These socks made me want to take them for a spin. Could I walk? I was convinced I could.

"Normally, if someone was this sick on ICU for, say, two weeks, it would take them two months to recover. Laurence was sick for weeks and weeks but then within days he was sitting on the edge of the bed and he basically was trying to run. He was just trying to get up and we were like: Oh, my God, sit down. You can imagine it's so dangerous. He's got all these lines in his neck, lines going into his arteries and a catheter; all these things that if you pull out you're going to cause a big problem but all he can see in his mind was like, 'I'm ready to go. Get me going.'" *Amelia Palmer*

The physios did small things with me during the day that felt like climbing Everest. One day they had me sitting on the edge of the bed. I was able to kick my legs out which made them very happy. One of them said it looked almost like a martial arts type move but I was a way off jiu-jitsu. Even lifting my legs felt Herculean. After that I was so tired the team put on a sailing programme and let me rest. The next day I did some more sitting up on the edge of the bed. It took such a lot of energy and strength to manage. After that the nurse put a martial art's programme on YouTube and then some sailing races. In the evening, she put on the BBC *Big Night In*. I was stuck in this hospital so it felt fitting but still beyond my comprehension was the understanding that everyone else was stuck inside too.

At night I seemed to get a second wind. The nurses on the late shift reported how often I would try to get out of bed during the small hours. Sam Morfee talked to me about how she would have to nudge me back in. She said I was quite determined. Apparently, I called her bossy and we both laughed. She said I had a good sense of humour.

I was only able to call Sam bossy after I had been fitted with a speaking valve on 26th April which enabled me to talk. When I first came round there was a hole in my throat from the tracheostomy. It looked pretty gross and was quite shocking. They put a speaking valve below the hole in your throat and you are making a noise, but you don't know how you are making it.

There was a bit of tube coming out of the hole and that is how I was breathing. There was nothing coming into my mouth or nose as that was patched up with a big plaster. The tube went straight into my stomach. That is how I was fed. Water is also coming through the tube so I had not been swallowing at all. I wasn't able to. Your brain and body just forgets how to use that area because it has been isolated. You don't know any of this when you are first coming round though so it just bewilders you.

Talking turned out to be a real struggle even with the valve in place. Unbeknownst to anyone then, part of my vocal cords had been damaged. I had a lisp. Half of my tongue was semi-paralysed and my lips didn't work properly, so I couldn't form a word with any degree of efficiency. Maybe I could have done some pretty scary voiceovers for movies.

My voice was very soft so I got frustrated when the staff couldn't understand me. Regardless, as soon as the staff gave me my phone back, I started trying to make phone calls to friends before I was compos mentis. Martine told the doctors I was a very strong-willed character.

"They gave him his phone back before he was fully recovered and there were so many messages from people wishing him well, sending love and support. Yet, he wasn't aware he had been in a coma for over five weeks. He had no memory of being on life support, none of the struggle he had gone through, none of the pain. The hospital didn't have any mental health nurses available to explain to him what had happened. To help him understand he had been unconscious for so long, that his body had fought so hard to survive. I was terrified he would read the messages from his friends, all hopeful and encouraging and still not fully grasp just how close he had come to losing it all.

Later, we found he had written some messages himself before he had any understanding of how seriously ill he was. It was heartbreaking, knowing that while everyone else had been watching and waiting for him to pull through, he had no idea how much time had passed, how much had changed, or how close he had come to the edge. The reality of it all hit me harder than anything else." *Martine Penn*

Looking at my phone confirmed the date and when I'd been admitted. It started to sink in: I really had *lost* the whole of April. Where had it gone? That was troubling but so were the very many text messages from certain friends and emails from work. Martine was worried I was getting distressed by them. Mischa deleted some of the messages using my iPad. She didn't think I needed to read some of the more extreme ones.

It was funny how some people reacted to my situation. Were they really reacting to me or was it more about them trying to navigate their own feelings during a global pandemic? I was still feeling pretty out of the loop concerning any of that. One of the nurses said that as soon as I could talk, I asked her if we could go to the pub. She explained that due to the COVID-19 outbreak all the pubs and restaurants were closed.

What was going on out in that wide world outside the hospital was still far beyond me. I wasn't even sure what was going on *within* the hospital, in the ward, or even inside *me*.

Chapter 14
Ta-da!

Now I was able to talk, if still quite weakly, I wanted to converse with the people round me. I wanted to understand what the nurses were going through because I really like to get people talking. So, when I was starting to become more and more awake it felt a bit like having a first strong coffee of the day, your brain suddenly goes, "Ta-da. OK? Yeah, I'm here now. I want to know what is going on out there."

One of the nurses told me, "I've not seen my husband or my son in nearly three weeks because I've been working here and I can't take it home, so I'm isolating in a different part of the house." She said, "But this weekend I'm seeing my family and my son's cooking for me. He's making prawn cocktail, mini burgers and apple crumble."

I remember that very clearly, because I was just fascinated by food. I wanted food. Real solid food. What I so wanted was some actual solid food. I can't say that enough. I just couldn't stop thinking about loaded cheesy pizzas and stacked greasy burgers. I wanted some real dirty food and a coffee. Every day I would say, "Can I get a coffee?"

Although I'd woken up now, I still had a tube up my nose feeding me into my stomach. And although I thought I was thirsty, they had saline water dripping into me. They were constantly making sure I was OK and improving.

*

As you're weaned off sedation and make progress, things

start to appear more real, more human. There was a constant buzz of chatter around me and about me; it was difficult not to be overwhelmed. One of the nurses washed my hair and it felt fabulous. Very considered decisions have to be made to remove feeding tubes, catheter, fluids and other lines but I did seem to be doing well. They removed the tracheostomy tube on 30th April. That is called being decannulated. I now just had oxygen coming in my nose, which is starting to sound almost normal, isn't it?

The dark month of April ticked over into May. When I looked in the mirror, I didn't recognise myself. The nurses were washing my hair periodically and sometimes I'd get a shave but my hair had grown long and I was gaunt and dishevelled. I was, however, smiling more and looking less puffy apparently. I also needed to use the air mask less and less. The physios were getting me sat up in a moulded wheelchair which was a positive step towards walking … if not an actual step yet.

*

On the first day of May I was given back my own clothes and helped to dress. I had a T-shirt on and some shorts. I sat up listening to my iPod which felt a bit more familiar. I was still getting confused though and I thought something had happened to my father. When I FaceTimed with Martine, she said he was well and my sisters had been checking in with him every day. That was a relief.

With the speech valve and my raspy, Barry White on fifty Cuban cigars a day voice, I asked if I could have food or a coffee. I was allowed some warm soup and some mash. Oh my God, how difficult was eating! It seemed a superhuman effort to chew and I was advised to slurp the soup and try to swallow this in small mouthfuls. As I had been on a ventilator for so long and then had a tracheostomy tube inserted into a hole in my throat, the SALT team (speech and language therapists) were advising me on how I should try to eat and drink for myself. The speech and language therapy guy started coming around and saying, "How are you doing?" And I'd try to speak. I'd squeak something out. Still work needed there but at least I was now talking without the valve.

My nose and my lips were in an absolute state though as if I'd been on a terrible winter holiday and not used any lip protection. The nurses had come around and put a toothbrush in my mouth to try to get some moisture on my lips but they were still feeling pretty shocking.

On 2nd May I managed to brush my own teeth which the nurses said after a month in ICU was a great achievement.

"It was definitely a relief to see people like Laurence turning the corner, because I think that was a big thing initially with putting a lot of effort into trying to save people. A lot of the time in intensive care historically, we would be managing people with lots of medical problems beforehand. People like Laurence, who was normally fit and well, it's relatively rare to actually look after these people on intensive care and so helping to get someone like that better is obviously quite a big, big thing." *Dr Luke Hodgson*

Given how my case was unusual, particularly before COVID-19, the team wanted to get me signed up to another research study. This one was regarding recovery. It looked at how patients could be supported in getting better after they had left ICU. The team knew that there would be a cohort of patients in a similar position to me at this time and it was an opportunity that was a bit too important to miss.

The doctors were predicting in conversations with Martine that it could be months or even up to a year for me to physically recover. For my cognitive dysfunction to fully improve could also take some time. It was all still uncertain but participating in another research study could really help the hospital to discover the most effective ways of supporting patients.

Many patients struggled after being discharged. When there are NHS staff constantly around your bedside motivating you with their tireless encouragement it is easier to do the things you need to do to improve your own health, but what would happen when these people were quite suddenly not there?

Chapter 15
One step at a time

While I was in the bed, I was just imagining that I could swing my legs out and walk somewhere. I was shocked to learn that wasn't the case. Having not used my muscles for such a long time they needed building back up again. You just can't comprehend that you can't walk. I'm thinking: this just isn't me. The first time I stood up again was daunting. With no balance, no strength, someone was holding each of my arms for support. After that came walking with a frame with a physio either side of me and one behind.

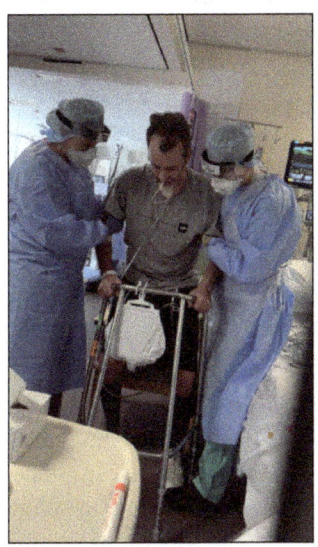

Figure 7

The physios were there at hand helping me with every move. They were having an *interesting* pandemic too. Unlike the nurses, physiotherapists rotate more when they are juniors so all physios have some experience of working on ICU. This meant that as the number of patients needing care soared and they were pulled in from different areas to help, most at least had some familiarity with the environment. They had varying degrees of experience but no one was being thrown into ICU as a complete novice.

They did, however, find

themselves dealing with things they wouldn't expect to under more normal circumstances. They also found themselves reassuring other members of staff who may have been redeployed to ICU without much experience. Physiotherapist Amelia Palmer said that sometimes it was a matter of being another pair of eyes. "We couldn't go in with a physio agenda and be like we need to do this with this person, this with this person, and this with this person. It was very much you go in and you just try and help wherever you can. And that might be moving someone, helping a nurse … that might be helping the doctors do something. I felt like we were just as much being physios as we were really just trying to be helpful because we were lucky enough in some ways to be people who were confident and competent to work in intensive care."

Gemma Stoner, another physiotherapist, felt there were things that felt like a whole new challenge, never experienced before in ICU in normal times. She added, "It was very different. We don't deal with drugs and medications normally, but then sometimes because we were around it every day, we became used to it and sometimes we were picking up on things that the nurses might not have picked up on because they're not used to working with patients that are so sick. You don't want to upset anyone or make anyone feel like they're doing a bad job but obviously just because we were used to working there, there were things that we might say, 'Actually do we need to do this?' or 'Does that need to go there?' or things like that." *Gemma Stoner*

Physiotherapist Jessica Owen said sometimes the physios could be a safety net. She remembers feeling valued for what they brought to the team.

"I think we were really valued as a profession during that

time and worked really well with other members of the MDT and in different areas. I think actually they really trusted us and wanted our opinion and they were guided a lot by us during that time as well."

She added, "A lot of us on Worthing ICU, we do a lot of the guiding on the tracheostomy weaning plans and weaning off a ventilator and we kind of lead on that in the Trust. And when people were going down to the ward, we were working on getting them home, so we were obviously working with other members of the MDT and the doctors and nurses on the wards as well." *Jessica Owen*

The team reflected on the differences with COVID-19 and how patients like me were in ICU for a much longer time than was usual and how shocking that was.

"People were really, really sick for a very long time. Obviously, you do get cases where people are really sick, but I just remember it would be days and weeks where this patient was the sickest patient you've ever seen in your career. And they weren't just like that for one day. They were like that for a week or two weeks." *Gemma Stoner*

She remembered how much oxygen I needed for days and days and the sheer frequency of the proning required for patients like me which had been unheard of previously. It was much more usual to prone a patient once or twice when they were at their sickest.

"They were sick for so long, you didn't know whether these people could get better. Were we going to get to the point to give them a tracheostomy to help reduce their levels of oxidation? Were we going to be able to rehab them? But they generally then turned a corner after much longer than we'd normally expect." *Mary-Kate Standing*

*

I may have been raring to take my first steps again but there was a practical matter that needed addressing. I didn't have any shoes.

"We try not to stand people up in ICU barefoot, because the floors are slippery and then [for that] the NHS socks are rubbish." *Amelia Palmer*

Apparently, Martine asked at this time if there was anything she could do. Amelia said, "Could you get him some trainers?"

"It's one thing to stand up in a sock or on a bare foot, but if you want to walk, you will need a shoe. Shoes are also needed for ankle support."

Martine got back to the physios to say, "Oh, my God. I've looked and all he's got is this brand-new pair of trainers he's never worn. Or he's got like, smart work shoes."

Amelia Palmer told her, "The thing is, whatever you give me will have to go in the bin. They won't let it come out of ICU because of the precautions.

Look, don't give me a brand-new pair of trainers. The smart work shoes are no good. What size are his feet?" Chances were he had the same size feet as my boyfriend. I said to him, "Have you got an old pair of trainers I can take to work?"

He had this old pair of Converse, "Yeah, absolutely, take them."

So, we put Laurence in these Converse. I'm not sure he would have worn Converse, but ... Those were then his shoes to do his rehab in."

Later Martine would write to Converse to tell them the story of the ICU, COVID-19 Converse shoes that meant a great deal to my rehab. Converse sent a voucher and Amelia ended up buying herself a swanky new pair of Converse.

By then she'd already replaced her boyfriend's pair ... or 'Converse-Man' as I came to call him.

So, with the Converse boots on and an ankle support fitted to my left foot, with Amelia on one arm and Gemma on the other it was all systems go. After tons of encouragement, I'm standing ... hold on, what the f*** is going on with my left leg? My brain was sending messages for it to move but they weren't getting through! We did five sit to stands. It was then suggested I walk but I couldn't. I was so knackered. I started to feel frustrated with myself and I sat back down quite heavily. One of the nurse's filmed the whole thing. I still have it. I look back at myself now. I was so disappointed.

Chapter 16
The imaginary toilet and other stories

There was a room in ICU. In normal times it was another room for treating people with a different disease. It's an isolation room but I was convinced it was a toilet.

"Can I just go to the toilet?" I would croak in my new craggy dialect.

They'd move to wheel in a commode chair.

"I want to go in there. I can get myself in there, can I go in there?"

It would never happen, of course. I was just dreaming I could hop out of bed but no, bless them, in they'd wheel that nuisance commode chair. I was still connected to oxygen and various monitors at that time and I'd have to be manoeuvred onto the chair. I'd sit there straining and willing a motion ... nothing would happen.

Then the poor old nurses would come and wipe my bottom as if I was a baby again. I found that so difficult to deal with. It was so frustrating not to be able to do something so basic. I wasn't worried about a lack of privacy because they'd always whizz the curtains round. I'd be propped up in bed, trying to work out why I couldn't use *that* toilet.

I was still coming and going in this dream space. I still believed we were on the beach and just outside that window was the sea, the sand, the seagulls, the fish and chips, the bracing salty sea air. In my head, I'd constructed this whole thing. In reality, I'm in Worthing hospital.

It wasn't until that last day, on leaving ICU that I realised there was no door and no sign to the beach. No ski resort, no much yearned for toilet. It must have been my brain's coping mechanism, filling in all the space, filling in all the time.

*

In bed number one on ICU, I was checked over several times a day and finally on 4th May the decision was made, I could leave ICU for real.

"Great! Where am I going?"

It was a momentous day. I was officially considered to no longer need intensive care. I was starting to get sparks of the *me* I think I used to be. To celebrate I walked across the ward with the help of a rollator frame. Nurse Sam Morfee said I was now moving onto "the homeward stretch."

It turned out it was rather a big deal for many others to see me leave ICU. I was visited by people I'd never seen before who said, "I saw you when you came in. I'm a junior consultant. You did fantastically well."

I'd nod and smile, thinking what did I do well? What did I do? Regardless, I thanked them for helping me. I imagined it was what a famous film star might feel when somebody out of the blue comes over, "Oh, I loved that … what you did there." And they're probably thinking I'm just doing my job – you didn't see the seventy-five takes it took to get that one.

*

On that last day in ICU, they told me they were going to move me but before they did there was one more thing I asked them to do. Weigh me.

Although I had grown to hate bed number one during my many dream travels, I couldn't deny it was an intelligent piece of kit. It moved in every direction. It heated. It cooled. It was very impressive, even if I had longed to get out of it so intensely.

So, who else would know how much I weighed but the raft I'd been lying on? They checked the bed and the bed spoke. It said, 68 kilos. 68 kilos?

"I weigh eighty-four to eighty-five kilos," I said, "You're sure that's right?"

Maybe the bed had a bug. The staff did a bit of calibrating and read it again. "Oh no, that was wrong."

Phew.

"It says sixty-two kilos."

What? Where has me gone?

*

Being discharged from ICU was very strange because everyone was really kind, coming to see me off, but then I was put onto a new bed and pushed out into a totally different environment. My transfer was onto a much larger ward called Beckett. It was an ordinary open ward in the hospital. It was so different to where I'd come from that adjusting to it was daunting. Rather than there being more staff than patients, in this ward there were many more patients than staff. There was a real mix of patients. I'd guess somewhere in the region of thirty to forty people. The coughing, the hustle, bustle of nurses attending to patients and the general commotion was a massive sensory overload!

I took in the surroundings and the other patients around me and assessed they were not in a good way. That was putting it politely. They were all in a state of recovery like me, some no doubt also from ICU. Did I look like that? Probably. Probably they were looking at me and thinking I hope I'm not in as bad a state as that guy.

You don't really get a chance to make any acquaintances in a place like that because everyone has that look about them, you know, like: What the hell am I doing here?

You waved at people. Sometimes they waved back. Some just gave you the thousand yard stare.

The noise was non-stop. I could hear other people suffering, coughing and groaning. I couldn't sleep and I became very agitated and anxious. It was horrible. I looked round at the other people and realised I was indeed like them: damaged and needing desperately to recover. I remember the guy to my right having an awful time and then the curtains went round. To this day, I'm not sure what happened. It was just one of those horrid daily occurrences during the pandemic in a hospital, I hope he pulled through.

I was in a really bad place in that part of the hospital because I couldn't go anywhere without an oxygen tank and a bottle. If I wanted to go to the loo, it was up to me to go for a pee because the catheter had been whipped out. I had to get my metal frame with its wheels, get the oxygen tank, clip it to the frame and then shuffle off to the toilet for nothing to happen. Not a major one anyway, just a pee.

Suddenly you go from being in ICU to being in a normal area. It was a real change from the attention of one-to-one round-the-clock nursing. You feel more alone, uncertain of what you're doing.

The nursing staff on the ward seemed very different. This is not a criticism, maybe they were contractors or temps brought in to cover the COVID-19 times; I wasn't sure. I did know I couldn't swallow anything particularly well, so all the drugs they'd been giving me in ICU they'd been injecting into me. When a nurse on the ward tried to give me these ginormous pills to swallow, I said, "I can't do that. I can't swallow that. My throat feels like it's the size of a pea." She didn't seem pleased with me and went away.

You could say I made a fuss. I felt awful about it but literally, within a few hours, I got moved into another ward called Beacon. How appropriate … a beacon of hope.

Chapter 17
The famous four on the third floor

Looking out of the window it was like the movie *28 Days Later*. It was just deserted. It was eerily quiet. There was no traffic. You could hear a lot going on in the hospital, but nothing going on outside. Life was lacking, no hubbub, no hullabaloo; the hospital was the noisiest place around.

We were three floors up facing south. I could see the sea. It really was a long way from that door!

That was the first time I'd seen daylight for a long time. There was no outside world on ICU because there were no windows that I could see out of and I'm not sure if they were real or imagined anyway. Seeing outdoors again motivated me. It was beautiful out there. It was May and it was really warm. The UK was experiencing a heatwave but no one could really get out there into it, well, not for any more than an hour of daily exercise anyway. Although, I didn't really understand that yet, so to me it was like something out of a sci-fi film to stand at that window wondering what was going on out there.

Getting to the window was a decent challenge. From my bed to the window, it felt a fair old way because I'd get up and walk as if I were inebriated. My left leg had suffered nerve damage; my left foot would just flop (the technical term was: foot drop). It wasn't much of a foot anymore when walking. As I tried to take each step my toes would drag on the floor, so the physios put an attachment into my Converse boots to keep it rigid so that I could still walk around, if in a rather ungainly manner.

You think, OK, is this me now? Is this what I'm living with?

When I felt them slipping into my mind, I tried not to dwell on those questions. I'd replace them with thoughts of getting home. I had my mission. I wasn't going to get distracted by a self-pity party.

I was visited by so many amazing NHS people. The feeling of that overwhelms me still. Every single person I came into contact with was so impressive, their passion for their work, their compassion, their patience, their selflessness, the sheer hard work and dedication. I was so utterly grateful. In my mind I was thinking of inviting them all to a huge party in their honour.

Beacon Ward was so much quieter; I managed to sleep. There were only four of us in there. To the left of my bed, was a hospital porter, a bear of a man, sixty-eight years old. Sitting up in bed bare chested, he gave me a beaming smile, "Alright mate?"

In the corner to the left of the room by the huge window was a fit seventy-two-year-old, an ex-kayaker for GB. And opposite me is a thirty-year-old. I learnt that all of these guys, and the people in the previous ward, were COVID-19 sufferers too. So many of us. I remembered the guy opposite from ICU. From pictures I've since received he must have been in the fourth bed and I remember seeing him being treated. In my dream state it looked like he was performing some kind of puppet theatre. He turned out to be really funny. All he wanted and was willing to eat was custard.

He had us in stitches because he just didn't give a damn about anything. He'd often try to get out of bed and his gown would fall off. Completely naked underneath, everything would be there for everyone to see. He still had his catheter installed so the other three of us, as soon as we saw him getting out of bed, we'd reach for our alarm buttons because we thought, Oh no, he's going to pull it out!

It was a different environment in Beacon Ward to the larger Beckett Ward. It was more like being back in ICU. The care was different. I think they'd worked out, all four of us weren't quite right or ready. All ex-COVID-19 patients, we'd also all been ventilated. The porter had been about three or four days on a ventilator. The kayaker had been on there for two weeks. I'd been in my coma the longest, though I didn't realise it at the time. I just felt we'd all been through the wringer.

We had our own private bathroom between the four of us. Showering was a major task. I'd sit on a special chair to wash. That hulking great oxygen tank was still attached and by now it felt like a third limb. I'd look at myself in the mirror in the bathroom and think, bloody hell, what's happened to my face? It was so thin and pasty pale, very weird to look into the mirror and not recognise myself. My hair was long. I was growing a scraggly beard and I seemed to have too much skin for my face. Each day I'd have a shower, shave and just try to be alright. To feel like me again. These were the small wins I celebrated in my mind.

Several times my general health and recovery were discussed, along with mental health and PTSD. A consultant visited me and I was asked to complete cognitive tests, like drawing a three-dimensional cube, reading a passage of text and answering questions on it, and some rational and reasoning questions. Maybe because I was *still* in a state of denial and not comprehending what my body had been through, I was very matter of fact about the tests and the discussions around my state of inward health. I was shrugging my shoulders and thinking just get me home I'll sort myself out then.

*

When the Physios called on me, they started by getting me to do more sit to stands. This is where you sit in a chair with your arms crossed touching each shoulder, so you can't use your arms to push yourself up. Initially, I managed about five. It's bloody hard!

Then we were off in a wheelchair to do a walking beep test, which was much the same as a timed shuttle run. You started at a very slow shuffling amble and attempted to walk about twenty yards round a cone and back to where you started. When I walked it felt again as if I was drunk. I wandered all over the place. My left foot and leg weren't responding in the way my brain was instructing them. Very frustrating. Not one to give up, I tried, as best I could, to speed up as the beeps quickened. I'm not sure how far I managed but it was knackering. There was also a small set of fairly steep stairs which we were taken to a couple of times a day to stretch out our legs and try to get our lungs working again.

The physios were brilliant. They were in every day. Not giving us a chance to be still. They wanted to keep us moving. As well as this, the physios were getting us reoriented and offering emotional support. With the amount of exercise and movement, they upped the ante. They were relentless.

"Laurence went into a bay where a lot of the other patients had been on ICU and also had that experience, so a lot of them had been extremely sick. It was just a matter of rehabbing them and getting them stronger. When people have been in hospital for a significant amount of time, especially up on ICU, we have a thing called our ICU pathway. Patients get followed up post ICU discharge. We set outcome measures when they're about to leave the hospital: a walking test and some strength testing – grip strength and some standing exercises. When we got around to doing Laurence's tests, we were doing a couple of other people on that day as well, and they were all egging each other on and going, 'Oh, we got this!'" *Jessica Owen*

Jessica added, "It was a really nice rehab environment that we developed down there, which was really lovely because I think a lot of them were extremely motivated to getting back to what they were doing previously … I don't remember talking much about the psychological effects all of them had but I think they felt like survivors. I guess we probably saw them as that too because at the time this was all a new thing. You see them up on the [ICU] unit and you think, this does not look good, and there were lots of conversations of: they're not going to do well … and questions: are we heading in the right direction? We're now having to prone them and we're having to do this. And then, all of a sudden you see them on the ward and they're walking and they're talking and they're improving and I felt a lot of the time you were just in awe to think: three weeks ago you were really not OK, and now you're here and you've survived."

Physiotherapist Gemma Stoner added, "We did see a lot of people survive and that felt good because all you were seeing on the news was people dying, but also, we were seeing a lot of people dying in ICU as well, so it gave a bit of hope that not everyone was dying. People were getting better and once they turned that corner, the rehab was actually quite quick compared to patients that we might have seen pre-COVID-19 who had been on ICU for a long period of time. They actually did regain a lot of function quite quickly."

Amelia remembered, "I think there was a lot of lovely camaraderie in that bay between the guys, a lot of encouraging each other, possibly to the dismay of the staff, to the point that it was like, 'Oh, my gosh, that's not safe.' You know, egging each other on: 'Oh, you can do that!' and 'Take yourself to the bathroom!' or 'Oh, I'm going to do a dance.' They were being a bit risky with their showing off to each other but that was also very Laurence, I feel.

Even later, when he came to the outpatient clinic, he was like, 'Oh, I think I'll try running.'

'Oh, my God, I'm not sure you should.'" *Amelia Palmer*

Chapter 18
I would know that fully PPE protected person anywhere

Staring out the window on Beacon Ward made it only too real that I had not been outside in over a month. In my previous *existence*, before COVID-19 and the coma, I'd be outdoors every day. I missed fresh air on my face, basking in the sunshine, the sounds of birds chirping away in the trees, so when one of the nurses suggested I be taken outside for some sun in a wheelchair, my answer was a resounding, emphatic, "Yes!" What a great idea. The wheelchair was brought in. I was manhandled into it with a large canister of oxygen strapped to the chair. Then we were off, wheeling our way through the hospital. We even went down the green lift because I'm now coronavirus-free, don't you know?

It still seemed I was in some bizarre world, which I was constantly challenging myself to assess, "Is this real?" I asked myself. "Am I really awake?"

The enormity of what I'd been through had simply not hit home. I was just not able to comprehend why and where and what had happened. Then with a *boom* we were through a set of double doors and outside. It was sunny, warm and I could smell the air. It was almost too much of a sensory overload. They wheeled me to a sunny spot, along a path that would normally be buzzing with people. The nurses left me alone for five minutes to close my eyes and feel the lovely warmth of the sun …

It was a beautiful feeling.

It was, however, over way too soon. We made the return trip back through the lower floors of the hospital, up the lift and back to the ward.

The whole sublime experience left me knackered and overjoyed at the same time. I had tasted freedom and boy, was it sweet? I wanted to go home.

*

I told Martine, I'd been sitting out in the sunshine. I told her how I'd sat there like a prize cat basking in the warm rays, just waiting to be bundled up in a *cat-napping* and whisked away. In my mind a plan was hatching.

"Maybe you could meet me in the car park, if you were wearing full PPE they'd just think you were a nurse," I said. Had my dreams given me this idea? In them, I'd seen Martine pose as a nurse before. Some things I was happy to not move from my dreams into reality but this might just work.

*

Call me old fashioned but on the day of my next outdoor outing I became even more determined to evacuate my bowels. I was convinced I'd got a month worth of excrement in there and I wanted it out. What was for sure is I had not passed a poo in the more traditional way for well over thirty-one days so I asked a nurse if there was anything that could be done.

I said, "I really need to go."

"No problem, Loz," she said, "I'll get you a laxative." She returned with a small tray on which was placed a latex glove and a suppository. "So just pop that up and away you go," she said, all smiles.

"Um, how long will this take to work?"

"Could be two hours or could be twenty minutes," she

said, still smiling.

All I could say in reply was "OK, thanks." And with that she was off to look after other people's needs, leaving me staring down at the answer to my pending need to evacuate my bowels.

I shuffled with my Zimmer frame to the bathroom, accompanied by my trustee bottle of oxygen. I got myself into the required position and inserted said suppository. Back I went to my bed, tank in tow.

Not too long as it goes! I was aware of a gurgling sensation and the strong need to fart. Dare I allow a fart? I did and immediately regretted the decision.

"Oh shit!" Quite literally. With the oxygen in place, I scrambled as best I could to the frame and got to the bathroom. I locked the door and positioned myself on the loo to commence one of life's simplest and, for many, daily occurrences. Boy, did it feel absolutely wonderful. Now, if the Guinness World Records ever wanted to look into world breaking poos, then mine must have been a contender. Crikey! It was like a Mr Whippy machine. It just wouldn't stop.

Several flushes later there came a-knocking on the door. Turned out the physio nurses were here for me. "We need to take you outside now."

"Yeah, be there as soon as I can!"

*

"At the time, bringing things into the hospital was not considered a problem, as patients who had Covid or who, like Loz, were now considered to have immunity from recent exposure couldn't be harmed and staff would be wearing PPE at all times. Patients and visitors were made aware that anything that came in would have to be binned unless it was easy to wipe/ decontaminate like phones and tablets. I believe all Loz's clothes from ICU went in the bin?! And similarly, we had people send in photos for their relatives to have by their bed, we had to only use digital copies or relatives agreed that they understood the photos could not come back out again afterwards.

Martine was extremely careful and isolated herself for an amount of time before she met Loz to be sure that she was not unwell in any way. I recall at the time she was very vigilant about ensuring everything was clean and wrapped carefully but we were already reasonably assured this was an airborne virus that travelled by human interaction and not via textiles. She was wearing PPE as were the staff and we were all outside. The rules at the time were: no visitors, but I think it was reasonable to make an exception for Loz who had been so long from his family and so unwell. As members of staff, it always felt hard that we were able to come and go but families weren't. To be shown via video link the person you love, on a ventilator while staff who are nothing but eyes and a mask, try to explain what's happening and reassure you. It must have been so awful for Martine, so arranging for them to meet was a good decision.

I remember Loz in the wheelchair, still physically and mentally weak. He was trying to be upbeat and forward thinking but it was a huge deal for him to meet and speak in person to Martine. Even though Loz was getting much better, I recall that he was still muddled sometimes and got tired and still needed oxygen. He was very unsteady on his feet and needed to rest a lot. He had lost a lot of weight too, so for Martine he must have looked like a shadow of the person that left nearly two months before to be admitted into the hospital." *Amelia Palmer*

*

I'd like to say I was exhilarated to sit in the sun again but I have to admit my thoughts were rather preoccupied with: do I stink of poo? Do they know what an amazing experience I've just been through? I was of course, elated that the plumbing was in order. I wanted to shout it through the corridors. On second thoughts, maybe I'd keep that to myself.

Bham! Through the double doors and we were outside in the beautiful sunshine once again. Only this time there was someone at the end of the path, dressed up in all the PPE gear. Impossible … but there was something about the way this figure was standing. I'd recognise that stance anywhere …

Martine recalls, "Before I went to the hospital, I meticulously washed my clothes in antibacterial wash. I even cleaned the clothes I was bringing for Loz and sealed them in a bag in the freezer, even though there's no real proof that would help. But it was something I *could* do, and I needed to do something.

We arranged a time. The nurse said someone would meet me in the garden since I couldn't go inside. I told her I'd make sure the clothes I wore and had brought for Loz were disinfected and I would be too. I had been in isolation for well over a month, completely sealed off and was wearing full PPE, like the staff.

It was such a big deal. The whole journey there felt surreal. The drive was strange, silent and eerie. The roads were completely empty. We were in lockdown, of course, but still … it felt like driving through a ghost town.

When I got there, I was early. The car park was full, but only with staff. No visitors allowed. I was wearing a homemade mask, one sewn by a neighbour who was making them for charity. I felt so out of place, so unsure of everything.

I sat in the car for what felt like forever, frozen with emotion. It was the first time I had been to the hospital where Loz was. The first time I'd been anywhere near the place where he had been fighting for his life – alone – for over a month. The weight of it hit me all at once. Eventually, I walked to the garden where I was to meet the nurse. I handed over the clothes and then – unexpectedly – she handed me some PPE. I put it on, still unsure what was happening.

Then, I saw someone being pushed in a wheelchair.

And then there he was. Loz. Seeing him – really seeing him – my stomach was churning. It was really him. He was alive. He was *really* alive. I wanted so desperately to throw my arms around him, but I didn't want to break any rules. I asked, quietly, 'Can I hug him?' The nurse and staff stepped back. That was my moment. My window. We embraced. I was overwhelmed. In my head, I kept repeating: Keep it together. Let him see you're OK. Be strong. Be the strong one.

Even now, I struggle to put into words what I felt in that moment. As much as I wanted to run and hug him, I had to stay in control. I had to be strong, for him. I held myself back.

Then, breaking through the emotion of that incredible reunion, Loz said, 'I'm so sorry, I stink of shit.'

And we laughed. We just *laughed*. It was such an incredible release. All the tension, all the fear, all the worry. It just came out in laughter. The nurse came over with a tissue, thinking we were crying, but I said, 'I'm so sorry, we're laughing.' That's us. That's *Loz and me.* Our humour has always been one of the most important parts of our lives. It carried us through this moment, like it has so many others.

He was so thin, skin and bone. I could feel it even in our embrace. But he was there – *my* beautiful husband. In the flesh. Dressed. Alive. He looked so pale, his skin almost translucent, and his hair had grown and curled in a way I hadn't seen before. I was stunned by how much he had physically changed. Of course it made sense: weeks in ICU, sedated, fighting for his life. I had been so focused on surviving each day, staying strong, getting through it all. I hadn't prepared myself for what survival would *look* like. And in that moment, the reality of it finally hit me." *Martine Penn*

As I got closer, I could feel a lump in my throat; my eyes were welling up …

It was my beautiful wife! I couldn't speak. I just wanted to hug her.

We embraced and a tide of emotion hit me. Martine and I, together again. We were both so giddy. Finally, I could touch, feel the person who means so much to me. The person at the epicentre of my survival. None of life's problems or worries existed for me in that moment. I was just so happy, so pleased to see her. She looked wonderful.

We stayed in that hug for a long time but all too soon I was flagging from the emotional bombardment. The nursing staff sensed it and wanted to take me back to the ward. They took the fresh clothes Martine had brought me, the reason for her *stopping by* which I hadn't fully comprehended.

Martine responded, "When I saw him for the first time again in the hospital garden, it was emotional beyond words. After he went back inside, I lingered there, trying to take it all in – and that's when the nurses began to come out. Not just one or two. So many of them. They came to see how *I* was doing. To talk, to offer comfort, to connect. These were the same people who had been fighting for his life just days earlier, who were still working under impossible pressure and, yet, they made time for *me*.

As I stood there, nurses introduced me to others passing by: staff arriving for their shifts.

'This is Loz's wife,' they said, with such warmth and care.

It was humbling. It was more than kindness. It was humanity at its most generous.

To this day, I still struggle to find the words to thank them. How do you express gratitude for something like that? How do you thank people for not just saving someone's life, but for holding space for *yours* while it felt like it was falling apart?

I will never forget what they did for us. Every single one of them. Their compassion, their strength, their quiet bravery. I carry them with me always." *Martine Penn*

*

The emotional toll of seeing Martine, a toll I would pay for again and again, had affected me. I was so grateful for the brilliant surprise but when I was left alone again on the third floor, I started to feel incredibly guilty for what I had put my family through. For what life must have been like for them. What a terrible fuss I'd made of this illness. Believe it or not, I was still operating in some kind of denial about what I'd been through. Only time would reveal all the information for me to digest. One fact that still haunts me to this day, is that during my stay in Worthing Hospital, forty-seven days, due to COVID-19, 150 people did not make it out alive.

*

"If anything, one of the common themes that I remember from those [ICU follow up] clinics, particularly from that first wave, was that there was a lot of survivor guilt. So, [survivors] were grateful they were alive and that they had done so well, but then they almost felt guilty about what had happened to other people and why they should have been the ones to survive. I really felt there was a lot of psychological processing that survivors went through about the trauma of what happened to them with this new pandemic. No one even knew what was going on. They were whisked into hospital with no friends and family support, like you would normally have … And then coming out the other side and wanting to be grateful that they had survived, but also being quite hideously traumatised about what had happened. But then feeling like … I can't feel … I shouldn't feel bad. I should feel good because I've survived and everyone's saying, 'Oh, you're so lucky, you're amazing.' And them feeling like: I don't feel lucky, I feel traumatised." *Amelia Palmer*

Chapter 19
Are we nearly there yet?

Seeing Martine reminded me even more of my mission. My ultimate goal was to get home by hook or by crook. By now I could use my phone. I could text. I could phone my wife, which I did a lot, chatting with her, video chatting with her and my daughters. So many texts, emails and messages were also coming in from friends and family. It was great but I still wasn't home.

I kept asking, "When can I go home? When can I go home?" Like a kid on a car journey: Are we there yet?

And the NHS healthcare professionals were saying, "We've got a lot of work to do before you can go home. We've got to know you can eat, walk, everything."

I remember they would come into our room to see us at least six times a day: checking oxygen levels, taking a blood sample … all that sort of stuff. And this is where I got sneaky. I'd worked out a way of virtually hyperventilating, so I could try and get as much oxygen in me as possible for the allotted time. If I timed it just right for when they were going to come in, I could try and get my oxygen count up.

Was I trying to cheat it to go home? Yes, but such is the motivation in wanting to go home. It was quite a tortuous process because I kept telling them I was fine. I was ready to go home!

Then one morning they said, "Yeah, you'll be able to go home today."

I thought, fantastic. So, I rang up my wife, "Yep, they're

going to let me go today."

"Great, what time can I come and get you?"

"Well, they don't know exactly when. I'll let you know as soon as I know."

So, I waited, "My wife's going to come and get me, can I tell her twelve?"

"We'll let you know."

The afternoon came around. The evening. The night. I was still in the hospital, waiting. Still not home.

"There's so much going on in a hospital for even one case and all the people involved have a lot of different opinions about: is he ready to go now? We need to keep observing him. He may not be there yet. One more day." *Amelia Palmer*

More than ten times each day I would say, "I'm ready to go home. Can I go home?"

On the day it finally did happen it was rather a surprise: there was no cheering or whooping. I got put in a wheelchair, with all my bits and bobs. I was given two bags of drugs, some nutrient shakes and a load of information. My wife was at the front entrance. She was expecting to come and help me out of the wheelchair but I did an Andy from *Little Britain*[23]. I stood up and walked to the car.

And that was it. I went home.

*

Martine remembers, "Back then, whenever someone survived COVID-19 and was discharged, hospital staff would line the halls and clap them out. It had become this symbolic moment of triumph, like you'd beaten the odds. But that didn't happen for Loz.

---

23 *Little Britain* was a BBC television programme created by David Walliams, Matt Lucas and Ashley Blaker and Andy and Lou were two of the characters: https://bit.ly/4lJeWjH

In the days leading up to his discharge, he would message me over and over again, saying: They're sending me home today. But every time, when I checked with the hospital, they said no. It wasn't true. He just *thought* it was. It started to feel like he believed I was somehow preventing him from coming home. As if I wasn't ready. Which was total rubbish. Of course I wanted him home. I had to constantly reassure him, 'I want you here more than anything,' I'd say. It became a daily thing, managing his frustration, calming his anxiety and hiding my own.

Then one day, around lunchtime, they said he might be coming home. *Possibly.* Finally, a sliver of hope. Later that afternoon, I messaged him and asked for someone from the ward to call me. They did. They told me they were having a meeting to decide, there were disagreements. Loz desperately wanted to leave, but they still had concerns. I told them, 'Please, just let me know either way. I need to be prepared.'

Around 5pm, Loz messaged: I can come home. Can you come and get me now?

I dropped everything, rushed to the hospital. There he was, sitting in a wheelchair at the front with one member of staff. I gave him a hug, grabbed his bags, turned around and he was already trying to get in the car. No fanfare. No clapping. Just this sense of urgency.

He said, 'Drive. Get me out of here. Just go.'

We were halfway home when the hospital called, 'You need to come back, we forgot to give you the tracheostomy dressing.'

My heart sank. I looked at Loz and said, 'I'm so sorry, but we have to go back.' He begged me not to. Absolutely begged. But I had to, I needed the supplies to care for the hole in his neck.

We went back, got the dressing and finally made it home."
Martine Penn

Chapter 20
Home is where the hard work is

Well, that was a bit of an anti-climax. You're telling me! It was.

On the journey home I was reminded of the scene from the first *Matrix* film when Neo played by Keanu Reeves is free of the matrix and sitting in the back of the car saying, "I remember that place. Really good noodles."

In the past few weeks my mind had created a whole new set of surroundings and realities that I now had to reassess. Some things I needed to accept were not real and I had to let them go but I was reluctant. They'd kept me alive and they still felt real. Even to this day they *feel* real.

It was the ride in the car that felt bizarre, I hadn't experienced the motion of driving or being driven for some time and the roads were empty. Martine explained what lockdown meant. As we sped along, I could see the evidence out the window; travelling through Worthing and back towards Thakeham it all looked so serene, quiet and *utterly deserted*.

As we pulled up to our house, it all felt so familiar but it also felt like I was experiencing it for the first time. It was surreal. Mischa came out of the house to meet me. I wanted to stand independently and to hug her but I needed to be supported.

"Mum went to the hospital and picked him up and it was weird just watching him walk up the driveway, up the stairs, looking like the tiniest, skinniest man I've ever seen."
Mischa Penn

*

"Mischa was waiting at the doorway. They reunited. It was beautiful, but Loz was completely drained. Just a few days out of ICU and now I, alone, and inexperienced was responsible for his care. I didn't know where to begin, I was surprised he wasn't discharged with any medication, instructions on fitting his leg brace or which size or way his tracheotomy dressing was supposed to fit. He could barely walk, couldn't speak properly, was very shaky. His thin, pale face with unhealed wounds across both cheeks, a scar across the back of his neck, his lower lip and tongue still dented and numb, his shaky hands struggling to raise a fork to his mouth and then he would dribble and not be able to swallow so he would spit the food out. His face looked thin in comparison to his mass of curly hair, I had to watch a man who a couple of months earlier was super fit and healthy, now he looked … haunted." *Martine Penn*

*

Normally you would just walk into your house, right? We've got six steps up to the front door. I would have bounded up these. Now they looked more like Everest. As much as I'd longed for this moment, I discovered the practicalities of getting *inside* my own home would be yet another mission. One I wasn't sure I had the reserves for, having just spent them on hyperventilating my way out of hospital. Thankfully, Martine and Mischa helped me into the house where I sank immediately into a chair.

From a now, thankfully, seated position, I took in my surroundings as my youngest daughter surveyed me.

"None of his clothes fit. His shoes didn't fit. He had lots of very baggy clothes on. That was odd. To be honest, he just looked awful: very skinny, grey, wrinkly, odd hair. Bless the nurses, they'd tried to give him a haircut, a beard shave, but done an awful job. So, one of the first things we did was give him a nice haircut ... *that* turned out to be awful too, but it *was* a haircut." *Mischa Penn*

*

Prior to going into hospital, I weighed a healthy eighty-five kilograms. When I left, I weighed around sixty. Most of my muscle had disappeared. I couldn't walk properly due to the dropped foot. My left leg, from the knee down to my toes, was numb and unresponsive, so walking felt very odd. I would have to almost throw my left leg forward and hope my foot would flop into place. I became out of breath doing the smallest shuffle/ walk. I couldn't talk properly. I had developed a lisp where my tongue had been pushed to one side to make way for the ventilator tube and my voice was very weak and reedy with no power. If I tried to raise my voice, it cracked and disappeared. I had a collapsed left side vocal cord and my throat felt really tight and narrow. And I had no clue who I was.

I was still struggling to comprehend what I had been through. Sitting in that chair and being aware of how much my body had changed and how alien it felt to me, I knew I was struggling. The words of the nurse speaking about mental health and PTSD played on my mind. Would I ever feel as I once had? Would I ever feel myself again?

Chapter 21
My second-best bed

Climbing the stairs and seeing my bed for the first time in nearly two months was very strange. Although I'd waited so long for it, that first night's sleep was not brilliant as I was so used to constant noise and light. I found it tough getting to sleep with the comparative peace and quiet of home. The thing I'd craved so very much was here, right in front of me, around me – my home – and now it felt extra-terrestrial to me. Everywhere you go there you are.

I surmised that if everything else wasn't from outer space, it must be me that had crash landed. We've got a big mirror in the bathroom and when I looked into it, I saw this version of myself I didn't recognise. What had happened to the rest of me?

Mischa remembers how I was mentally struggling to process everything. How it was too much for me to take in for a period of time. I was desperate to figure out what had happened. Apparently, I had been convinced that I was in Wales while in hospital.

"It took him a while to adjust, but it also took us a while to adjust as well. We were trying to make him healthy food. Bless my mum, she said, 'Right, he's out of hospital, let's make sure we get him some good food.'" *Mischa Penn*

*

"The next morning, my phone didn't stop ringing. Nurses, doctors, nutritionists – all calling with instructions.

I'd made Loz vegetable soup, thinking: healthy and easy to swallow. To be told, 'No, he needs protein and fat to put on weight. Make cottage pie, the fattiest meat you can get, cheese on top.'

I don't cook but I tried. For him. I made the cottage pie. Loz, normally king of the kitchen, must have found it frustrating. But he was grateful.

Then he said something simple, something heartbreaking, 'I can't swallow mashed potato.'

That moment really hit me. I was so grateful to have Loz home. I had been warned that his recovery could take up to eighteen months and I was ready to help in every way I could.

Beneath the relief, I carried a quiet fear – knowing that when the full weight of what he had survived finally hit him, it might not just be his body that struggled to heal, but his mind too." *Martine Penn*

*

"The doctor called to check in on him, 'Right, how's he doing?'

'He's eating well. We're making him some healthy food.'

And the doctor's like, 'No, no, stuff that man full of pizzas and burgers. Get that man fat!'

'Oh, all right, OK. I guess we're going to McDonald's tonight, Dad.'" *Mischa Penn*

I was in the background cheering.

Only I found, when I did come to eat the fatty foods I was craving, my eyes were far bigger than my stomach. I would think, sure I can manage a whole pizza or a burger and chips. I'd eat maybe a quarter of it and then be absolutely stuffed. My stomach had shrunk so it made piling on the pounds considerably harder.

The nutritionist was saying, "He must eat more!" The weight wasn't going on quickly enough. "If he can't eat, he's got to drink the shakes."

Out of nowhere huge boxes of shakes began arriving. They were packed with nutrients and vitamins but the taste took some getting used to. I had to do three a day and that was a real struggle. Eating in general though was such a chore. I seemed to have a type of eating trauma. If I had a mouthful of something, I had to have a cup of hot water next to me so I could sip it. I'd have to get the bite all mushed up in my mouth, before I could swallow.

With drinking I would have to take a breath and *then* drink. I couldn't just gulp it down. And even then, I still had quite a few choking and coughing incidents. The unconscious competence of eating and drinking is really something not to be taken for granted.

Mischa said it was as if she was having an out of body experience to see me looking so very weak and under nourished. She saw a different side to me. No longer the man of action she was most familiar with.

"It was an odd feeling because it wasn't like it was Dad. I felt I saw a different side to who I thought my dad was, then you finally see that people are actually very vulnerable, very weak. It was like a different person all over again. My dad and I had always been very close growing up, and we did a lot of stuff together. We did jiu-jitsu together. We shot together. I was basically a son for him. Still am.

Your dad's supposed to be the one to protect you, and he is the man of the house. I felt then, not that he was weak, but he just looked so frail. I think it changes the perspective of what your dad is at that point. Not that I don't see him as that now, but more so I feel: I want to protect you and I want to look out for you." *Mischa Penn*

Being very tired, very run down, Mischa remembers made me quite short tempered. For the first couple of weeks I was obviously, to her, feeling very ill.

"It was weird to adjust to, but it was also nice to know he was home. So, there was a huge sense of relief, but also a sense of: we're not at the end yet. We made a conscious effort to keep positive spirits in the house." *Mischa Penn*

It wasn't always easy for my family to know what I needed or how to help. Mischa remembers it being a matter of just cooking dinner, giving me time, letting me adjust and letting me tell my stories and ask questions.

Sitting in that familiar chair once again I finally took stock … That was when I realised the catalogue of what wasn't right with me. Only when I got home did it finally *hit* home. What a state! There were so very many things I would have to relearn and to say that was daunting was an understatement. My life had utterly changed and there was no way it would ever be the same again. I could have sunk into a depression in the armchair and never got up again.

Thankfully, the NHS again proved to be fantastic. They wouldn't let me rot in that chair, even if I'd really wanted to, which I didn't really. I wanted to be well. It's a challenge though, as a human, to wrestle your short-term desire to wallow in exhaustion, with the long-term goal of being able to manage the steps into your own home without feeling like you have to have a few hours kip afterwards.

It really does make a big difference to get you out of that chair when people are looking in on you and reminding you you've got to get better. Every day a district nurse would come in dressed up in all their PPE suits. Everyone was still taking this pandemic very seriously, which was good because

I didn't want more like me, struggling to relearn how to live.

For me, everything I've done in my life has been around performance, peak performance, managing people to do and achieve things through leadership, so I had to take my own medicine. I had to relearn how to learn, so to speak, and that was huge. I felt impatient as I struggled with things that *should* have been easy for me to do. Relearning *how* was massively frustrating.

The physiotherapists kept encouraging me, "Laurence, you've got to take one day at a time." They were checking in on me too and the team could see my step count each day via the Fitbit the hospital had given me to monitor my recovery. They gave me an exercise plan and it was literally: sit in a chair, stand and then sit back in the chair. Five times a day. Well, so far, I'd got the first bit down.

My Fitbit smartwatch measured my step count but also my heart rate. This led to a few interesting incidents in the first couple of weeks, when out-of-the-blue, it seemed, flashing lights would appear.

*

"I called Dr Tim Fooks to let him know the good news, Loz was home and to ask for some advice. That even though we fortunately have a downstairs bedroom, he recommended that if Loz can make it upstairs it would be better that I am beside him in the night, should he need me.

Loz was at home, slowly recovering. It had been a few days – maybe a week –but we were taking it day by day. He'd started experiencing heart palpitations, so he rang the GP. Thankfully, our local surgery was still open, operating as a COVID-19 hub while so many others had closed.

Our GP happened to be in that day. He said he'd see Loz straight away, but told him to wait in the car park rather than come inside. After the examination, he warned us: if Loz had another episode – especially with his heart – we needed to call an ambulance immediately.

A couple of days later, in the middle of the night, Loz woke me up. He didn't say much, just looked at me and said, calmly but seriously, 'Call me an ambulance.'

Every day, I had been monitoring him religiously: oxygen levels, temperature, heart rate. That night, when I tried to check his vitals, the machine flashed up: ERROR. That was it. No hesitation. I picked up the phone and dialled 999.

It was harder for me this time. So much harder. I truly thought we were out of the woods. He was home. He was recovering. We'd made it through the worst, hadn't we?

When Loz said, 'Call me an ambulance,' I felt the floor shift beneath me. My stomach dropped. The last time I'd made that call, I'd thought he'd be gone for a day or two, get some oxygen and come home.

So, this time, when I reached for the phone, it wasn't just about the moment, it was everything coming back at once. The fear. The helplessness. The trauma. It felt like we were being pulled back into it all over again. Like the nightmare hadn't ended after all.

Thankfully, he came back the next day. Relief flooded me but it was short-lived. Not long after, the hospital called and said he needed to come back again. Another check on his heart. Another round of anxiety.

He was on a strict recovery diet. I'm no chef – not even close – but I had a big meal planner, trying to keep things on track. It wasn't exactly gourmet, but I was doing my best. Lots of protein. That morning, he hadn't even had breakfast before we had to turn round and head straight back in.

And for me, in that moment, it just felt endless. Like I was stuck in some cruel loop of fear and uncertainty." *Martine Penn*

"Dad being Dad didn't tell us his heart rate was over like 190, or something ridiculous. And blue lights are outside at f***ing 3am They've flagged up that his heart rate is going crazy. So, things like that happened for the first couple of weeks. He thinks that he's OK … Suddenly an ambulance would just turn up and you'd be like, Oh, *OK!*" *Mischa Penn*

In those early days home, the paramedics came a few times to check me over. My body was still in fight mode, adjusting to being back from the hospital … or as it had deduced from an unknown source, Wales.

Chapter 22
Two sits down, one stand up

When you leave hospital, there are so many benchmarking tests that you do. Yes, there was the stand-up, sit-down as many times as you can in a minute. I think I did about twenty-five, something ridiculous and I was absolutely exhausted. I have to say, I was buggered. Then you do a grip test with these two devices and that apparently is an indicator of your whole-body strength. These grip things measure the amount of pressure you can put and it was not very good. It was like a seventy-five-year-old/ eighty-year-old man grip, sort of thing. And various other things, lung function tests and that sort of stuff, and then you're off.

The physios gave me this whole exercise plan and some of the exercises were just literally hands up in the air, sit in a chair, stand up and sit down ten times and then get to thirty and then get to sixty. Get as many as you can in a minute. And they were constantly trying to challenge you to do it. For me, I was going to do it. There was no two ways about it. I was going to smash it.

Beyond what I was given, I set myself little goals. I was privileged to be able to draw on my own previous training in fitness, which really helped. I wanted to get back to where I was and try and go past that.

After a while, the physiotherapists upped the sitting and standing per day. They then slowly started to introduce other exercises like lunging on your legs to get them working again and introducing weights to start rebuilding muscles.

They did some horrible tests at a specialist unit in Haywards Heath. A nerve specialist stuck long hollow needles into my left shin area and also my foot area. She then inserted electrodes inside the tubes into the flesh, sending electric pulses to see if the nerves would respond. She seemed able to hear what was going on. I could feel this odd sensation that to be honest was starting to make me feel like throwing up, but my big toe suddenly moved!

Eventually she said, "They are responding, but it could be eight months or even eighteen months before you get full use of your leg and foot."

Eighteen months!

I couldn't move my big toe. I'd look at it and will it to move with all my might but ... nothing. It felt like it was dead. Sometimes I'd feel a bit of pins and needles in it but not much else. All my muscles had atrophied. My biceps had gone. My bum had disappeared. And that's just because you're lying down for so long not doing anything. You're not expending any energy on movement. You're just literally wasting away. And I suppose that was a hard thing to deal with.

"The muscle mass loss is huge because normally you've got a lot of reserve, haven't you, from getting around? But all the muscles just wither away, essentially. It takes maybe a few months to get back to what they were beforehand, so all your body systems are not working as they should for some time." *Dr Luke Hodgson*

*

There were a lot of calls about mental health. Often. "Are you OK?" or "Do you need any help?" and, "Do you want to speak to anybody?" You hear so much in the news about a lack of help with mental health. I would have to disagree with that from my experience. It was offered and proffered.

However, despite the help, it was a good three weeks of me just being dumbfounded. Still, not really able to come to terms with where I was. I couldn't even work out where I had been, but whenever I felt like giving up there was someone there to pick me up again and refocus me on another body part to work. Although it was really hard, it gave me a new appreciation for my body and all the things that needed to align to keep it functioning well.

Every day, a district nurse would turn up and check me out and then a physio would turn up and say, "Right, we've got some exercises for you." They really went to town on my leg. They gave me these amazing set of exercises to try and get it going again. And they didn't relent. They didn't relent at all. They then said, "Right, yeah, we can't get you back to hospital but we're going to set up a Zoom session with the speech and language therapist."

This fabulous speech and language therapist called Samantha would appear on my PC and stick her tongue out and ask me to copy her actions. I couldn't go in to see her as we were still in lockdown, so I was sent a Zoom invite and that's how my first consultation started.

She talked me through why I had the problems and devised a set of specific exercises, showing them very close up, starting with sticking my tongue out and trying to move it left and right. It felt like an unresponsive lump of rubber. Really odd and thick in my mouth.

Having started to eat solids again, I had inadvertently chomped on it a few times. Jeez had that bloody hurt! Samantha would say, "Right, these are the exercises you need to do with your tongue."

She also gave me all these vocal exercises actors and

singers do so it might reactivate my vocal cords. However, even with the exercises, Samantha was getting concerned. They needed to do some investigating to see what was going on, so they stuck a camera up my nose which was rather gross. It went up my nose and down my throat and while it was up there I had to repeat after Sam, "The king's coming. The coming is the king. The king's coming."

She could see on the video that one of my vocal cords was moving and the other one was not.

Sam said, "Look, there's the problem," pointing at the stagnant chord. "What we can do is we can operate on that and we can put a filler in or you can just give it time and see what happens."

I didn't need to think for long, "I'll give it time and see what happens." No more operations, thank you very much.

The tracheostomy had basically paralysed part of my vocal cord which now wouldn't move. So, Sam gave me some more exercises to see if we could get it going again. If you imagine the noise a horse makes … you have to hum quite violently while doing that. Different ranges, different levels of pitch and you vary that while doing the noise.

As weird as it was, it worked. My voice gradually returned. I couldn't shout still because when I'd go to say something and put some volume behind it, my voice would just collapse. It is a hard thing to wrap your head round trying to shout, "Hey." And it goes *squeak* … and just disappears.

The quality of my lips improved with all the stimulation, so that was an added bonus. The Ear, Nose and Throat (ENT) people had meetings with me online too. They said, "Don't cough."

When you're swallowing, if you cough then it doesn't do your vocal cords any good. Coughing would aggravate what was going on there, so I had to resist the temptation to cough and learn to swallow.

Chapter 23
A bit Fitbit

Getting home, my life became, in some ways, simpler. I had only to focus on a series of goals, small steps that added up.

Eating – gain weight and relearn how to swallow.

Walking – work on my dropped foot with the physios and get my step count up.

Talking – participate in speech and language therapy for my semi-paralysed tongue and paralysed vocal cord.

Get strong – do the exercises and push the weights.

That was my list. Still, I'd got to keep everything going to stay on track and for a good month after I came home, my life revolved around regular monitoring. Midday and in the evening, I'd take my blood pressure, check my oxygen levels and log my heart rate. I had to do my blood pressure the old-fashioned way but now you can get devices that go on your wrist. I had a blood pressure machine and an electric thing where you put a clip on your finger that shows the oxygen levels in your blood.

You can go a lot further with an app. You can log what you're eating, even what you're drinking. Are you drinking a litre or two litres of water a day? Do you fall short? You just had a coffee … anything like that could go on there but I didn't log the dietary stuff. Instead, I wore the Fitbit I'd been given back in the hospital and did the exercises.

While I was in the ICU, you may remember that Dr Todd Leckie came to see me and said, "We've got this trial. We'd like you to wear a Fitbit for twelve months, so we can see how you do in recuperation. We want to track your recovery. What do you say?"

I'd made a commitment to myself and to the NHS. How ever I could help them. I was going to help them, because I was just so fascinated by how they go about mending and looking after people. They don't care about your height, weight, race or sex. They just care about *you*, whatever and whoever you are. I said, "Yeah, absolutely. I'll do that."

Dr Hodgson, the senior consultant in ICU and a crucial part of the team, who saved me from the darkness of that coma, was also involved with the research study[24] into supporting once critically ill patients in their recovery using wearable technology.

"We know that at least twenty-five per cent to, I think, about forty per cent of the country, don't do as much activity as the basic WHO recommendations for activity levels. So, we already know that a lot of people are less active than they should be when they're well, but it's doubly important to try to be healthy if you've been ill or if you've got an illness. In all walks of life, whether it's before an operation or after an operation or you've just been admitted very unwell to intensive care, trying to optimise how somebody does activities is very important. And using technology like smartwatches can be a way of doing a combination of things, like nudging a person to help them maintain their activity levels.

Using baseline and increment in activity is effective. It's associated with all sorts of good outcomes. So, people live longer, they're less likely to have all sorts of illnesses: cardiovascular illness, strokes, diabetes, all sorts of chronic conditions can be improved. But I think in terms of using it

---

24 https://www.ncbi.nlm.nih.gov/pmc/articles/PMC9063865/

in healthcare, we still don't really fully understand the best way to use the technology. So that's partly why we try to get people into research studies to better understand what's the most effective way of doing something."

I now like to call Luke, the 'Fitbit Guy'. I'm not sure how he feels about that. For me though, wearing the smartwatch worked well.

As soon as Dr Todd Leckie gave it to me, I put it on there and then. I wasn't sure how to use it yet but over time I managed to get my head around how it worked. If you haven't seen one before, a Fitbit isn't very big. It just sits on your wrist and it can tell the time, but it's also counting your steps. If you start doing more exercise, it will recognise that. You can click it and say: I'm having a gym session, or I'm having a walk or a run. It measures your heartbeat too. There's also a green light that's measuring your blood oxygen levels.

Wearing the device gave me something to focus on that I had agency over. That I could see changing. The hospital team gave me the same login that they also had access to so the physios were able to look in and adjust my recovery plan where needed. Physiotherapists like Gemma Stoner were on the other end looking at the watch data to see, "OK, how many steps is he doing a day?"

"We have a study going on [with] one of the consultants where we were giving out smartwatches to see if it aided their recovery or worked as a prompt or a goal setting. It relied on the patient syncing the Fitbit every so often, but we were able to see their step count and stuff. And some people were doing absolutely nothing and then Loz was up there ... with a ridiculous number of steps and exercise." *Gemma Stoner*

Physio, Jessica Owen remembered how my step count was beaten only by a porter whose job enabled his high number of steps. I have to wonder if that was my friend from Beacon Ward.

Mary-Kate Standing was very generous when she said, "Oh my God, Laurence pretty much rehabbed himself. Every time I'd be like, 'Oh, have you done this?' And he'd be like, 'Yeah, yeah, I've done that and more.' And then I'd be like, 'OK ... erghh ...'" *Mary-Kate Standing*

The truth is, the physiotherapist team were crucial in encouraging me and keeping me accountable.

"I'd give patients a phone call to egg them on and just see what they were doing. Could I give any more exercises? But, yeah, looking at some of their data it was insane how quickly they'd come on." *Mary-Kate Standing*

I was a very motivated person after I decided I wanted to get better, but for people who aren't necessarily motivated to do exercise this is where the Fitbit can really help to create a conversation and try to prompt people to engage with the process of recovery. Luke Hodgson explained to me how keeping in touch with people after they leave hospital can be a challenge. So, the goals of the smartwatch study, I was involved with, are to explore productive ways of doing that.

"We were looking at how to set people up with structured exercise programs to then incrementally do more but also be able to remotely see what they were up to, so having a sort of feedback loop between talking to the patient on the phone and seeing what they're doing. That seemed to work quite well and giving them some basic step count advice seems to be quite handy for a good proportion of them. We've been doing work in various other pathways with this sort of approach because giving people clear goals and plans are quite helpful, as opposed to just saying all you need do is to get active or something." *Dr Luke Hodgson*

If I'd been given a target of 10,000 steps out of the gate that would been quite a lot, so with the smartwatch data the team could build up to that by giving me appropriate goals for where I currently was. To begin with, my journey was just round the ground floor inside the house, and that would knacker me out. Then I managed to get round the garden. After that I roamed a bit further to the fields out back – the ones from my Richard Hammond-like vision. It meant a lot, being able to walk there every day. My intention was to get more and more of that land done in increments. Doing that for a while, I suddenly noticed I was starting to feel better.

For me, participation in the study had very positive benefits but running studies can be expensive. It's not so much the cost of the technology. Some smartwatches are relatively inexpensive. However, running studies is very expensive. You need the infrastructure, admin and research nurse time. It's all those sorts of things you've got to get funding for essentially. Dr Hodgson explained to me why rolling out a smartwatch to everyone wouldn't be appropriate at this stage.

"They're relatively expensive and you want to make sure you're doing something that's beneficial because there's always cost implications to anything. So, by doing research you can actually see, or discover, whether doing physical activity intervention using this technology versus not, does that lead to, for instance, better health related quality of life or stop the person getting rehabilitated to hospital? Does it make them more active? All these things have to be tested scientifically, so that's why we do the research." *Dr Luke Hodgson*

Besides the impact on health, the pandemic also saw advancements in the way we used technology day to day. That's also had an impact on the Fitbit recovery study.

"Obviously, there were lots of technological advancements that eventually came through, weren't there? All the Teams and Zooms, etcetera, are much more easily accessible and used in healthcare now. Whereas before, that sort of thing wasn't at all really. Telemedicine has been around for decades, hasn't it? But it wouldn't be routinely used in hospitals at all. You'd normally see a person in the outpatients. Normality became having phone calls with people you wouldn't normally do routinely." *Dr Luke Hodgson*

The other piece of research that Luke had been talking about was the possibility of an app that uses some kind of AI, which is available, to prompt that person to say, "Look, I notice you didn't get out to do your 5,000 steps or your 2,000 steps today. How are you feeling? Is there a problem?" and, "Go online and click this video that's available on your phone to show you how to do it ..." It would prompt you to try this, try that and monitor your progress.

"Someone like Laurence is very motivated and already was into the technology or exercise, but for a lot of people, that wouldn't be the same sort of thing. And if you've not got a family support there to help you it's harder. We know that about fifty per cent of people who've been admitted to intensive care get re-admitted to hospital in the year afterwards and it's something like twenty-five to forty per cent of people who are still not back to work after a year. A lot of people are still fairly incapacitated or they've still got ongoing problems in that year after intensive care. So, we know the aftercare is not fantastic. There's a lot more intensive care units that have these follow-up clinics these

days, but we put together ours during COVID-19, so the physios, the nurses and I all meet up together to see a patient in the follow-up, as part of a multidisciplinary team (MDT)."
Dr Luke Hodgson

My rehab would be very different to the next person but the app would understand that and give each individual the prompts they need. It would also encourage recovery linked to what we know about the connection between physical and mental health.

Chapter 24
Cornwall and heart

Two months of goals set and tests and goals smashed and I was starting to feel more like myself again. You know that in three months' time you're going to get another crack at the tests to see how you're doing, so I had that in mind. I wanted to prove I was a life worth saving.

In that period, I suddenly got my appetite back, piling the food in and even piling the weight back on. The physios gave me exercises that used my own body weight as resistance: press ups (on my knees to start with), sit-ups and burpees. All quite easy to me by my normal standards but it was up to me how I made it harder. They gave me loads of resistance, training exercises using big, gigantic bands, where you just put it round your legs and move that leg against the band. You can stand up, holding on to the back of a chair and just move your leg out sideways and backwards to reawaken the muscles. That's when you know the muscles are there. I could feel them. They just needed working, so I got some dumbbells and a barbell. I added weights and went at it.

It is fair to say a few times, I overdid it and just felt awful. I had limits but I wasn't always good at recognising them. Being unwell wasn't part of my identity. I had always seen myself as fit and healthy, so getting back to that space was everything to me.

Physiotherapist Mary-Kate Standing remembered seeing me at the three month mark.

"In the clinic it's myself, an ICU consultant and our critical

ICU nurses. We see them [patients like me] at three months and we review, to see how the patient's getting on. Chat to them about their experience, any questions they have, any kind of medical concerns they need to address, but also review those outcome measures. And I think he was up there with our best outcome measures. That's only three months after discharge from ICU, which is not a long length of time really, to face coming out of hospital into a different world at that point, to then try rehab, get used to normal ... what *was* ... normal life." *Mary-Kate Standing*

The team thought that considering gyms still weren't open and I wasn't going out much due to the restrictions, my progress was much more than they'd been expecting. The strict lockdown rules eased a bit as the summer went on and people were being encouraged to, for example, Eat Out To Help Out[25]. My wife took the opportunity to organise a trip to Cornwall in July. I think she thought a change of scene would do me good. We were all largely outside for mingling and social distancing of some kind was still being *advised*. Luckily, we were amazingly fortunate with the weather. We stayed at a place called the Stargazy Inn in Port Isaac. It was still quite chilly but we were sat outside. A young woman came out and gave us a lovely rug to wrap round us. We just sat there having a gin and tonic and reflecting over what we had been through. I looked out over the amazing scenery and thought, thank God. Thank God this turned out the way it did.

Looking back now, Cornwall was where I turned a corner.

Or at least I felt I had. When I came back, I had an episode. You may remember that when I returned from hospital, I experienced some fast heart beats and emergency visits from

---

25 https://www.bbc.com/news/uk-67658106

paramedics. Well, it seems the heart palpitations were not done with me yet.

When you think about it: May, June, July. It's not that long, really, not in the grand scheme of things. I wanted to believe I was back; I was all better. In a basic sense, I was at least on the mend. Only, my body had some other ideas.

These episodes are not for the faint hearted ... but for some kind of hearted which was still rather an enigma. During these events, your heart goes through some kind of roof. It would be sitting at around seventy beats a minute and all of a sudden it just jumps up to 170 and 180 beats a minute. And it's a startling, scary feeling because you can't stop it. Your arms and legs feel heavy. Obviously, you think, shit, I'm having a heart attack or I certainly did! But that's not right because then after five to ten minutes it just stops, leaving you feeling confused and on edge.

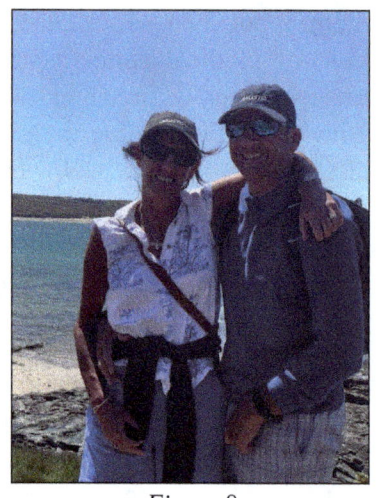

Figure 8

The first time this happened it maybe lasted a few minutes and I thought, well, it's nothing. I looked it up and discovered it was called: heart palpitations, or fluttering. The internet said you can stop it by bearing down, so you have to imagine you've got bad constipation and you're trying to squeeze something out. *That's* bearing down. There's a nerve called a vagus nerve running down the side of your neck. It's the longest of the cranial nerves and it carries signals between your brain, heart and digestive systems. I learned you can manipulate that. Alternatively, you can splash very cold water in your face and shock yourself, which makes you gasp. That can reset you.

These heart palpitations occurred another couple of times. I talked to my doctor and he got me down to the surgery, did an ECG test and said, "Shit, you've had a heart attack."

Using another machine shifted his diagnosis slightly.

He then did another ECG test and said, "No, you haven't. This machine is faulty."

There seemed to be nothing wrong with my heart at all. Perfectly normal, so it seemed. He did however suggest we do some further investigations, so I went down to Worthing Hospital where they did more extensive tests. Nothing.

They gave me a device to wear for twenty-four hours. It's stuck on you, down by your side, collecting data, so for a whole twenty-four hour period. It records your heart and then you drop the device off. Still nothing.

The doctor then said to me, "If it happens again, whatever time of day, call 999, get down to A&E."

I'm like, "OK, fine, it won't happen again. It's just a thing." And then three in the morning on a Sunday and *bang*! There it was again. As soon as it started, I checked my smartwatch to check and see if I could stop it.

No such luck. Half an hour later I went to my wife with my tail between my legs. "Can you ring an ambulance? My heart is still hammering away."

Ten minutes later and the flashing blue light appeared in the sky round my home once more. A couple of young paramedics had me in the back of the ambulance, trying to bite down on a pen. I tried everything but nothing worked. They put a heart monitor on and they could see it: 200 beats a minute. And this was forty minutes in, so it was down to Worthing hospital again, into A&E, so I could be hooked up to their machines. I was getting a bit of an audience now because they were astounded at what was going on with my heart.

My whole chest felt like it was beating so furiously, like an engine. I didn't feel I could do anything though because, was it actually pumping blood this fast? It seemed to be going nuts. This is a COVID-19 hangover[26]. I've now heard about this. It can be the result of a lot of different disorders around the blood, and the heart, and the lungs. Blood clots have been mentioned. The news about COVID-19 being responsible for blood clots was yet to really break when I was sat in A&E yet again, feeling a bit sheepish. There were some rumours though, just nothing conclusive as yet.

I remember the doctors saying to me, "Right, we're going to do this procedure; we're going to use a drug." They said, "What's going to happen is we're going to inject you. You'll feel a strong sensation. Your heart will stop and it will restart again."

And I was like, "Woah, pardon? Stop and restart again?"

They did it and literally the relief was amazing. Ah, thank f*** for that. Normality was restored straight away.

The team looked at my records, "So you were in here in May?" They couldn't work out why the episodes had been happening but thankfully it turned out to be the last time. Since the procedure, the drugs, the stopping and restarting of my heart, it has stayed the course.

"Anyone who's severely unwell for a month on intensive care, your whole body's homeostasis is disrupted, isn't

---

26 https://achievehealthcolorado.com/blog/12221/THE-COVID-HANGOVER

it? And so having arrhythmias and all sorts of issues, neurological problems, etcetera, they just go hand in hand with being very, very ill. A load of ladies started to worry because a month or two afterwards [after having COVID-19], all their hair started falling out. That's also where you get nail problems, don't you? Where you've had a trauma at that particular point and so that's what leads to the hair loss and so on. It grows back again." *Dr Luke Hodgson*

*

The body finds lots of ways of coping when you are severely ill; some of them aren't always helpful later. Long Covid was a term created in the Spring of 2020 by people experiencing ongoing symptoms after having COVID-19.[27] Some people, even with a much milder reaction to Covid than me, reported suffering long term effects. There were reports in the news of sufferers whose lives changed dramatically with their fitness levels plummeting post-virus. The causes of Long Covid became hotly debated. Was it a result of the virus's effect on the body or of the body's reaction to the virus? Were some people suffering from trauma-related fallout from COVID-19? Were my heart palpitations something similar?

My body had gone through a trauma and it is very possible the palpitations could have been connected to my body's coping mechanisms. You hear about people with chronic illnesses or back pain where the body anticipates trouble and reacts by contracting muscles or activating pain. Was my palpitation episode part of a trauma response? It seemed possible. However, the stopping and restarting of my heart did work, so whatever the cause, it did the trick.

---

27 https://www.ncbi.nlm.nih.gov/pmc/articles/PMC7992371/

Chapter 25
Training

As I continued to improve physically, the physios suggested I try the Couch to 5K running program. Now I can run, but God, do I hate it? I do. I'm not good at it.

I said, "I'll cycle." I've cycled before. I've got lots of muscle memory around it, so it was in those moments that the idea came to me to set a big, hairy audacious goal. The physios gave me the inspiration to do it.

A very dear friend of mine who has dealt with mental health issues and swore by the benefits of mountain biking, quoting that it literally saved his life. We made a pact, Tom [Simmonds] and me. I said, "Look, I want to do something for the NHS."

I think Tom said, "How about riding the South Down's Way in a day?"

"YES! Will you be my training buddy?"

Without hesitation, he said, "Yes, I will."

So that was that. Plan concocted. Goal set. We planned to start off training by getting to thirty miles, then forty miles, fifty miles and then finally to seventy-five miles. To see out our plan we'd just have to do the extra twenty-nine to the full 106 miles on the day. It always seems like a lot from zero but still, we had a lot of hope we could do it.

Once I set myself this super ambitious, probably foolhardy, goal of cycling the South Downs Way in a day, word started to spread. When the physios found out that I was doing this event I think they may have thought I was a bit off my rocker but to be honest, that training saved me. Having that goal gave me something to work towards and I made sure I set up accountability by aiming to raise money for the NHS as part of my ride.

To do so, I contacted the charity Love Your Hospital (now merged with East Sussex and called My University Hospitals Sussex). They raise money for St Richard's Hospital in Chichester, Worthing Hospital and Southlands Hospital in Shoreham. Their mission is: To enhance the care and experience of everyone who comes through the doors of our hospitals … "We raise funds for treatment, care and research which go over and above core NHS funding, making a real and tangible difference to patients and staff alike."[28]

I spoke to John Price who'd been working in the Trust for nine years and for the charity for nearly five.

"Easiest way to explain it is that we help fund anything from as small as something like a five-pound bravery certificate, so that might be for when a child goes down for a blood test, through to the biggest piece of kit we have funded, which I think was about 1.6 million pounds, for a robotic surgery arm, which helps with laparoscopy surgery. So, keyhole surgery where we don't have to open up patients, reducing risk of infection or longer hospital stays. All those types of projects and anything in between really that falls outside of government funding. We deal with pre-birth to post death and everybody in between; you name it, from a cut finger through to somebody who's got the worst possible diagnosis in the history of the world, that's where we deal."

To give you some examples, last year the charity funded Glideaway beds for family members to stay close to their hospitalised relative, three monitors for stroke patients, two

---

[28] https://www.myuhsussex.org/

ECG monitors to support cardiac patients, and heart shaped cushions for patients with breast cancer. I wanted to raise money for the ICU team that saved my life. John assured me the money I raised could be ring-fenced in order that it went to the area I wanted it to.

He remembered the first time we spoke.

"Laurence came to my attention when we got a phone call in the office. It was a gentleman saying, 'I've had COVID-19. I basically nearly died, and I want to do something to say thank you. And this is what my plan is ... This is what I want to do ...'" *John Price*

John listened to my story.

"When you actually hear he nearly died and had to learn to do things again ... that was an incredible story. And for the charity, let's be honest, it was a story we wanted to support. It was such an inspiration. A man who had been so fit and lived his life doing everything, pretty much, at the top end of what he wanted to do ... If he wanted to do sport or anything, he was pretty good at it ... but having to learn to do everything – ride a bike, walk, all those types of things – again, was just phenomenal. To hear that as a story and then he wanted to cycle the South Down Way was ... 'Yeah, we'll be right behind you.' It was a great story and a real privilege for me to meet Laurence and help support him in that way." *John Price*

The charity really helped me with setting up a JustGiving page and getting the word out.

"We gave him the basic tools, explaining about the JustGiving page, how to finance and how to get the story out there, but let's be honest, he was very active. There are a lot of people that need a lot of support. Lawrence didn't need a lot of support from us. He was very active around getting people on board and making sure people knew the story: the TV, the press, the radio, all those types of people. He was already doing that and didn't need me to do that. He was very much a proactive fundraiser, so we supported him with *silly* things like t-shirts and the JustGiving page and logos and wording around the charity and why he wanted to support us. Anything we could help with, post event stories etcetera. On the day is where I think we really came in, to make sure he felt that we massively appreciated what he did." *John Price*

And I did! As Tim Fooks said, "Charities were not having an easy time of it during the pandemic. I asked John a bit more about his own experiences at the time I was in hospital.

"Personally, my role in the charity changed. It was really a strange time in the NHS, because I ended up changing my role from a fundraiser because we couldn't fundraise, because there were no fundraising events as such. We're quite heavily based around events and people doing events for us and because obviously there was social distancing, people weren't getting together. They just stopped overnight, so our funding, as such, stopped.

We were quite proactive as a charity. I worked every day during COVID-19. We had a lot of people and there were a lot of unbelievable donations that people wanted to make to say thank you to the NHS because they were still working. I became pretty much a logistics manager overnight. I could tell you some of the most random things we had donated to the trust, to our staff members, but right away: 15,000 Easter eggs. We went through Easter so a lot of the shops and the supermarkets had Easter eggs that had been ordered because they were going to sell them. People like that went well: Actually, we can't sell them. What can we do with them?

Overnight, we were like, right, you've got 15,000 Easter

eggs coming in, one for each member of your staff, so you're trying to then think about distribution and storage and how to do that across 15,000 people. We were getting donations of hand creams for nurses and doctors, and also of masks and stuff like that." *John Price*

Part of John's role changed again when he became involved in rolling out vaccinations to front line staff. This ended up being around 50,000 vaccinations for hospital workers, police officers, fire crews, ambulance crews and carers at home.

"They were very long days and very late nights. We were open pretty much from seven in the morning through to ten at night. And then I'd go home, eat, go to bed, get back up and do it all over again." *John Price*

John is now largely back to his fundraising role in the charity. Like many charities, they have found the way people donate money has changed but John advocates getting involved as fundraising should be fun.

"At that point, always say the clue's in the title: fundraising. The first three letters. Make it fun. Make it something you want to do. OK, so you've got something you really like doing, let's think about ways of doing something like that because if you've never run a marathon before, don't turn and say: I'm going to run a marathon, because that's going to hurt." *John Price*

If you're interested in checking out the kinds of projects they get involved with or maybe have an idea of something you could do, please look at their charity website[29].

Once John helped me set up the JustGiving page online, I got to work telling everybody I knew. It gave me accountability.

---

29 https://www.myuhsussex.org/about–us/ see the QR code at the end of Bed Number One

I thought: I can't *not* do it now. I'm committed to this.

If I hadn't had all those things set up, it would have been tempting to just not see it through, but it just fell into place. It felt like the right thing for me to do. The plan came together really quickly. The healthcare professionals found out I was doing it, so invited me down to the hospital in August to do what's basically a test. They put me on an exercise bike, strangely enough, strapped up with heart monitors, a breath monitor, and then, "Every minute," they said, "We're going to increase the resistance on the bike. You can't stand up, so you have to stay sitting down and just go for it."

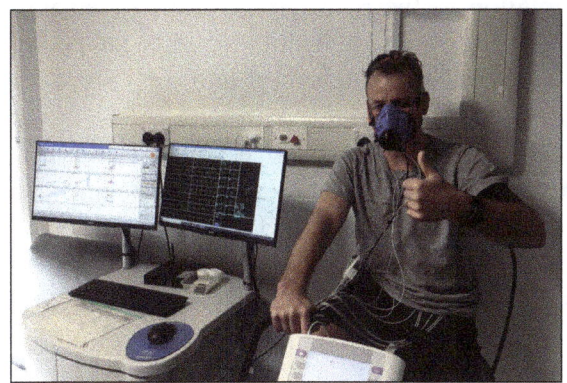

Figure 9

The doctor who was testing me was very young and he was almost yelling at me to keep going and go harder and go faster. After ten minutes, I was sweating buckets. I thought it would be easy but it was so tough.

Funny enough, Nicky, who was one of the nurses that saw me when I first came in, was there too. It must have been strange to see my transformation. What a journey! After the test, the doctor showed me all the stats and graphs and said,

"Bloody well done; you're fit!" He said, "I can show you these two graphs, the blue line here and the red line here. This shows me that you've got some significant scarring in your lungs. We would expect that for what you've been through."

I thought, OK, so I know that my lungs are challenged, but to keep them fit, I've got to *stay* fit. There's no ifs, buts or maybes.

I got invited again back to the hospital to meet the respiratory team: Dr Hodgson, Dr Leckie, Physiotherapist Amelia Palmer and another nurse called Nicola Bean. This was in relation to the research I was involved with. They said, "Right, we're going to do three tests today. We've got the grip test, the sit to stand test and we've got a walking test."

The walking test involved cones and a beep. I had to walk round the cones before the beep sounded, the timing between beeps got shorter, meaning I had to go faster at every turn.

I'm proud to say, I smashed the record for the walking beep test. The sit to stand was like, "Oh, my God!" I smashed that too. And for the grip test they were like, "Who are you? Who even are you?"

But they were really pleased to see me again and I kept thinking, well, I don't get why there's so much interest in me. I hadn't counted on how many people I'd never consciously met seeming to have a vested interest in me doing well. I was, of course, unknowingly a reflection of their diligent work. It was almost like a 360-degree recognition: This guy's bounced back! It made me all the more determined to raise money for the NHS with my epic bike ride. I had to make them proud.

All the pieces kept stacking up to make backing out of

cycling the South Downs Way in a day impossible. I reached out to somebody on LinkedIn who was working for ITV. In the email I wrote: I've got a story; would you be interested …?

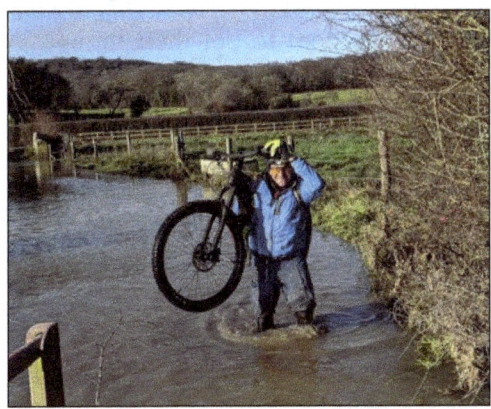
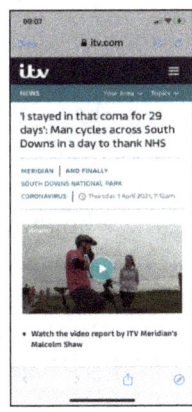

Figure 10 *Figure 11*

They came back a day later, "Yeah, we'd love to. It sounds like a really good local story. We'll make it happen."

Two guys from ITV Meridian turned up, an interviewer Malcolm Shaw and a cameraman. We had a conversation. They came to our house and they filmed a piece. During the filming we arranged to link up with Amelia Palmer live on a Zoom call. Getting it aired on ITV was pretty daunting. The pressure to get out there and start shaking the tin was mounting.

The JustGiving page turned out to be another unexpected boost. When you donate you can either be anonymous and maybe you might type: Good luck, mate, here's £20, or something like that. Or people could leave their name. For those who might be even more invested they could leave an email or send a direct message. Thankfully, a lot of people did that and a lot of people leaving messages were nurses.

That really stopped me in my tracks. It was very moving. Here I was, desperately wanting to do something to give back for all the care I'd received and here they were giving to me yet again! I didn't want them to put their money in there because this was in honour of them, and yet they did. It was so heart-warming.

I downloaded all the comments into a giant spreadsheet. I read through every comment. Some people, I really didn't know who they were. Some had just seen the story featured on ITV: Love your story, mate. Well done. Good luck on the day. Some were a little more *known*: I'm a friend of your sister; I'm a friend of a friend; My sister is a nurse ... and then there were those who had been a part of my journey, although I didn't always know it.

Remember back when I woke up in hospital and didn't have any shoes to wear to properly support my dodgy foot as I re-learnt to walk? Well, it was through the JustGiving page I met physio Amelia Palmer's boyfriend who'd donated his Converse trainers to my cause. I had finally met 'Converse Man'!

He signed off his message: 'Converse Man' ... so from that point on that was how I referred to him, while he referred to me as 'Jiu-jitsu Man'. This was the code Amelia had used at home because she was unable to reveal my name for confidentiality purposes. 'Converse Man' left his email, so I responded back to him: Hi, you must be the guy that was the owner of the shitty shoes? ...' I didn't really call them shitty shoes. It was Amelia who had originally said that when I made such a grateful fuss of them.

"They're just a pair of shitty shoes," she said.

'Converse Man' wrote back: My name is Rick. I'm Amelia's partner. I've heard so much about you.

Chapter 26
We're putting you on the board

There's a board up at the hospital. It's a thank you board of sorts. COVID-19 survivors from that first wave go on the board. The team have collected their stories, the ones they hear in the outpatient clinic about patients who've been in intensive care and gone on to really regain their lives post ICU. I'm on that board.

"That's something that's always a worry with intensive care, that you save a person's life, but they don't actually go back to living and a quality of life they want and consider acceptable. What is really nice with the outpatient clinic is that we do get to hear these stories and hear that people have gone back to really living their lives and they're happy and they're not debilitated. One of the physios made a board with lots of the stories and photos, which Laurence is part of and put it up in intensive care as a sort of positive inspiration for the staff, as well.

Morale got so low, seeing so many people die, you really needed those happy stories to remind you why you're doing it every day." *Amelia Palmer*

Fellow physiothcrapist, Gemma Stoner also reflected on the survival stories.

"Lots of them are keen to share their stories as well. About three times a year, we invite all of those previous ICU patients to … we call it WRAPS, Worthing Relative and Patients' Support Group. And we often have people that want to stand up and share their story and I guess reassure other people …

this is what I'm doing now." *Gemma Stoner*

WRAPS allows previous patients of ICU to reassure those that might not be as far down the line that they too will reach a similar stage. It helps keep people motivated on their journey. I went to WRAPS once and spoke about my journey and where I was now. I hoped it might inspire people. Gemma explained that the group wasn't everything it could be yet. Due to the pandemic they had to impose limits on numbers. Instead of being people that had been on ICU anytime in the last however many years, it was a group of people who had all had COVID-19.

I was thankful to be on the gratitude board but I was thankful to all the amazing people who had gone, in my mind, above and beyond to save my life and also my quality of life. There would never be enough I could do to express that feeling of immense gratitude towards them.

"It must have been soon after he came home, they brought in a massive box of goodies, like really delicious truffle chocolates and loads of wine. When we were allowed, a big group of us who looked after Laurence just had a get together and very much enjoyed drinking the wine they'd very kindly given us. That was obviously very much appreciated but also it was quite nice because the get together was probably the first time we'd all been together outside of work. It was in my garden, over a year after he'd left. And it was the first time we could get together without breaking any rules. No rule of six or anything like that. There were probably about ten of us." *Gemma Stoner*

It sounded like the party I'd wanted to throw for them when I was still in hospital. I was so glad to hear they had been able to have it. Amelia still remembered me talking about the party.

"All he kept saying was, 'Girls, we're going to have a party. We're going to have a garden party. When I get home, everyone can come round, everyone from ICU. I'm going to invite everyone to this party.' And we were still like, 'Laurence is a bit delirious. He's not quite in the real world.' And then, of course, we saw Martine, and he was like, 'Martine, I've told them we're going to have a party.'

And she was like, 'Ha, ha. I think maybe we've got other things to worry about for the moment, Loz.'

Meanwhile, he's inviting the whole of Worthing Hospital to a party at his house.

Then Martine subsequently said, 'Oh, no, I didn't think he was confused because that is exactly what Laurence would do. And he would have a hundred per cent meant, yes, we are going to have a party.'

But it was just funny that we sort of put that down to all the confusion, but he wasn't confused. He did genuinely want us all to come to a party, but unfortunately, that never quite played out because COVID-19 didn't disappear in the way we thought it was going to." *Amelia Palmer*

Chapter 27
Research champions

As we moved through the second half of 2020, it came to my attention that the NHS were looking for public and patient contributors with lived experience of being treated in hospital for COVID-19. It was another way I could prove useful to the teams that saved my life. I signed up to assist on an urgent public health panel. It wasn't like anything I had ever done before but if I could use my experiences for good, I would.

This was well before there was a vaccine available and it was vital that more was understood about how to roll out the drug trials in readiness for the treatment of COVID-19. I would get invited to a meeting on Microsoft Teams. Prior to that meeting they'd send me through the particulars of three or four different drug trials to read through. It was all confidential, so at the time I didn't know what the drug trials were by name. As time went on though, it would become a bit more obvious as drugs, vaccines and treatments started to be talked about more readily in the media.

2020 was shuffling on and as the days of the year drew in, things also started to go dark again with the COVID-19 situation. Lots of people were working on possible solutions so there were a great many methods being considered, including pills that could be sent to people so they didn't have to come to hospital, through to respirators. People like me were needed to be in on these meetings. Once I'd read the studies, I'd be asked: if I could take the drug in a trial, would

I take it? If yes, why? If not, why not?

Besides me, there was one other regular member of the public like me on these panels. I don't know if there were others but I'd often see the same person again and again. My partner in COVID-19 survival *crime* ... be it at quite a distance.

I would log on to the call and the screen would be full of pages and pages of people. As many as seventy doctors. It looked much like a stamp book. You saw some of them sitting in their respective hospitals. They'd have a stethoscope hanging round their necks and people walking past in the background, going about their business. I was thinking, wow, this is really happening right now. It made it feel so much more real. It was intense and fascinating.

Some of the doctors I'd even seen on various breakfast TV news programs. I recognised a blonde lady from *Good Morning Britain*. Professor Chris Whitty wasn't there but people beneath him were. There were people like Medical Director, Professor Nick Lemoine, who was the guy who chaired. He would brilliantly control the meeting. When you consider the amount of people that were there and data that was gathered it was incredibly well done. You had your bit to say and you knew at 7.10am they'd come to you, because there was always a pre-call before that meeting. It'd be his PA, or even Nick himself, and they'd say, "Hi, Laurence. How are you? Glad you're on board. We're going to come to you first tonight, so if you've got your questions prepared ..."

And I'd say, "Do you want me to run through them?"
"Sure."
I'd tell them the questions I had.
"Good, good. Like that. Great. Right see you at 6.45pm."

And then you'd grab a cup of tea, get prepped, then the meeting call would commence.

They would talk through all the studies. As I listened to what was going on, I'd realise my questions were pretty weak, because they'd already covered the answer ten times in all their answers, but I still had to go through with it.

My imposter syndrome was in full on mode but it felt like important work. This process enabled there to be some patient public involvement in the decision-making process, so some feedback could go into helping them create the trial before it went out to people who were needed to participate in the studies themselves. Sometimes we could be really useful by pointing out what was missing or where more information was needed to point out potential side effects or what to do in the event of side effects. Who and how do I contact if I have an adverse reaction? Etcetera." It was easier for us to see how they needed to make drug trials more *user* friendly.

Being involved wasn't only fascinating but it led me to being signed up as a research champion. Suddenly I was a voice of authority, as a first-hand survivor of this shocking illness that was rocking, frustrating and mystifying the world. Research is everywhere in the NHS. It's huge, but you see the struggles that the National Institute of Health Research and Clinical Research Network have because it's not understood enough by Joe Public.

When you hear health researchers what do you think of? Men in white coats, lab rats ...? In people's minds, when you say drug trial, they think of some poor rabbit or rat in a box being injected. This was not that. Sometimes it was just people electing to take the treatment themselves as part of a study (and mostly a blind study, in that out of a hundred people, fifty would be on a placebo and not the actual drug, but the participants wouldn't know who was taking which, only the research team).

In one study (led by a professor at London School of Hygiene & Tropical Medicine and a research fellow at THIS Institute) the team videoed me and other people who had survived COVID-19 after being in ICU. They took the stories of the people who had been through it and collected their experiences so that when we encounter the next pandemic, all the data gathered from the COVID-19 study will be available and will likely be invaluable to future research.

Whoever approached me from whatever part of the NHS, whether the CRNCC, the NIHR, the PPEI, QTIP, UPH, I said yes. They were throwing a lot of work my way. It wasn't paid but we did get any expenses covered. I wasn't in it for money though. For me it was about getting involved, giving back and trying to help slow the disease that had stopped me in my tracks.

The 44th Dimbleby Lecture was delivered by Dame Sarah Gilbert, the lady who created the first vaccine.[30] She was aware of what was going on in China with that first outbreak. She was observing, watching it and hatching a plan. Once, on 11th January 2020, Chinese scientists made the genetic sequence of the novel coronavirus publicly available online[31], Dame Sarah Gilbert and her team knew they could make a vaccine based on their previous work. However, when funding proved difficult to attain, she resolved to worry about how to pay for it later or else we'd all be paying in an even bigger way. Because of that decision, Dame Sarah

---

30 https://www.ox.ac.uk/news/2021-12-07-professor-dame-sarah-gilbert-delivers-44th-dimbleby-lecture

31 https://www.cidrap.umn.edu/covid-19/china-releases-genetic-data-new-coronavirus-now-deadly

Gilbert and her team came up with the first Oxford vaccine. I remember it coming through the trials, being part of it, that monumental change of fate.

It's hard to deny now that the development of the vaccines changed the whole playing field when it came to COVID-19. However, even after the vaccines were announced, they were still looking at other medicines for people who were pregnant or had diabetes or had existing underlying heart conditions that might react badly to one vaccine or another. They were continuing to try and get trials off the ground. The people with those conditions needed to try the drug or enter into a trial to try the drug, up to a point it was continual.

NIHR COVID-19 Understanding and Elimination-Trials Implementation Panel (CUE-TIP)[32] was the last program I participated in. At the end of the study I got a letter saying, "Thank you very much for your involvement. It has been very valuable," from Professor Nick Lemoine. Without members of the public to assist with studies, it wouldn't be possible to make progress. And research touches a very wide range of areas within the NHS. For example, there's a massive amount of research that goes into women who are pregnant, who go through various problems that could in turn affect the child. The more research they can get the better, so if you're working in a maternity ward, you'll be targeted by the National Institute of Research to sign up as many people who come in with childbirth needs to do research. It's not going to be detrimental to the unborn baby. They just want to know what you're going through so they can measure it. That knowledge is valuable.

Through being a research champion, I got another unique

---

32 https://www.nihr.ac.uk/documents/nihr-covid-19-understanding-and-elimination-trials-implementation-panel-cue-tip-terms-of-reference/28260

invite. Out of the blue, I was asked to be a judge for the *Nursing Times* Awards in the research category. When I said

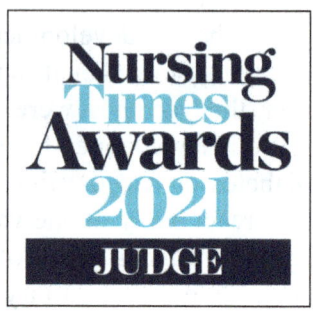

Figure 12

yes about forty packs came through, all were individual research projects for me to read. Each one was anything between three to twenty-five pages, including support and documentation. I had to read and then score it. Then I sent it off to be assessed. The other judges, all professors and very senior doctors, did so too independently.

From that process a shortlist was created. I was invited to London to meet and interview the nominees. It was the first time I'd been to London since 2019 and by contrast it was just empty. Some of the entrants came in physically to present, while some did it on a big screen via Zoom or Microsoft Teams because they couldn't get to London. We all made our own notes and then at the end of that day we concluded by noting our scores. Luckily, I voted emphatically for the lady that won. This was quite a boost for me as I was still questioning what I was doing there? And, how was I qualified?

Later that year there was a black-tie do in London Grosvenor Hotel, grand ballroom, hosted by Naga Munchetty and attended by over a thousand nurses, doctors, professors and a couple of Joe Public, like me. It was so heartwarming to see so many people representing and also supporting the awesome world of nursing. Watching the research category winner's reaction and look of surprise on her face was priceless.

Chapter 28
The South up and Downs Way

I accept now that weather-wise it would have made a lot more sense to make this epic journey in June, but I had a very specific reason for choosing 31st March 2021. It was exactly one year since I'd been put into the coma. That was one year to recover as best I could from the darkest days of my life. As luck would have it, we had great weather, no rain. It was still dark though when we set off from Winchester at just before 6am. Meridian, part of the ITV network,[33] wanted to follow the whole event and get it clipped up and on the evening news that day, or at least the very next, so I recorded a bit on my phone at about 5.40am.

As daunting as the task ahead of us was, we decided we were going to enjoy it. It's a beautiful route. An awesome route with 13,000 feet of climbing and consequently probably 13,000 feet of descending because it's up and down a lot of the way. It should be called the South Ups Way not the South Downs Way. Still, as gruelling as some of the climbs were, we reached a high point within the Queen Elizabeth Country Park where we grabbed a fuel stop of black coffee and cheese sandwiches. Once refuelled, we were looking down a very steep hill called Butser Hill. It looked challenging with lots of uneven looking ridges but with our usual gung-ho attitude we set off. At the base of the hill, we knew it had been bloody fast. We checked our speed readings … forty-one mph!

"We'll be there in no time." laughed Tom.

---

33 https://www.itv.com/news/meridian

We stopped roughly every twenty to twenty-five miles to refuel, keeping up the calories before we cracked on again. About fifty to fifty-five miles in, Storrington marked the halfway point. There's a car park right on the South Downs Way called Chantry Post. The TV crew were set up there in two places so they could film us approach. John Price, from Love Your Hospital, was there too. They'd set up banners and I could see them as we drew near. John and his colleague were dishing out bright red t-shirts, like the one I was wearing.

"He sent us his route and rough times for when he expected to be where, so we went up to Chantry Post. We tried to make it as visible as possible by putting up all the signs and all the flags. It was a beautiful day. My colleague, Denise, and I went up and supported from the charity aspect, but what was really nice was a lot of the guys that cared for Laurence on the intensive care unit had made the effort to go up as well. A lot of the nursing staff had

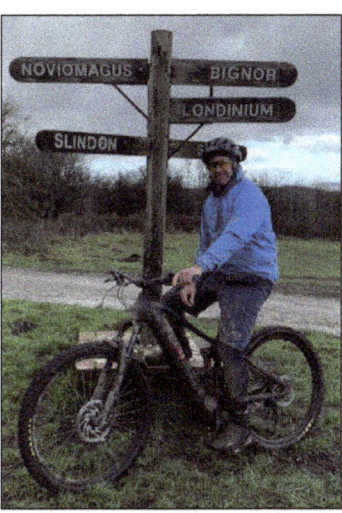

Figure 13

taken the time to meet him and cheer him along. To see them there was great because I think it really brought home to Laurence that what he was doing was really important. We did that as a charity to say thank you, but the nursing staff had taken time out of their day, whether it was a day off or whatever, to be up there and do that. That was really kind of fabulous." *John Price*

John remembered the really good view, which meant he could see us coming over the horizon and cycling up to them all. I have to say, I was feeling knackered as I'm sure Tom was. When I looked back at what I said to the camera crew, I now feel I could have said something more poignant …[34]

"I stayed in that coma for twenty-nine days, so it felt like a fitting way to put two fingers up to COVID-19 and to show what can be achieved with a bit of resilience and hard work, motivation, but also, I have to give massive thanks to the NHS. The staff that looked after me, they're amazing. They did a fantastic job."

Maybe it wasn't as poignant as I would have liked but I hadn't prepared for it and my attention was wandering to thoughts of food. I was also very aware of the people who'd come to say hello; in particular the group of nurses. I wanted to go and chat with them as soon as the interview was over. I spent some time speaking with these amazing people, all of whom had met me but I sadly didn't recognise them. It was truly brilliant to meet them all and typical of the selfless attitude of the nursing staff in the NHS. All superheroes to me.

John Price talked more about the impact of a thank you on the NHS team.

"That's the really important thing that I think people underestimate. Actually, the guys get a thank you and they love a thank you. Let's be honest, any bit of gratitude where somebody goes, 'Thank you. What a wonderful job you've done,' is brilliant. People come back to the hospital quite frequently to say thank you. And often, they will bring in

---

[34] https://www.itv.com/news/meridian/2021-03-31/i-stayed-in-that-coma-for-29-days-man-cycles-across-south-downs-in-a-day-to-thank-nhs

biscuits and chocolates. I'll be totally honest with you, I think the NHS runs on sugar. Often people will come back in with really nice gestures. It's great that they do but to do what Laurence did went so far above what an average person would do.

COVID-19 was a really weird time for everybody. No one really knew what was going on ... I think what he had gone through really touched a lot of people's hearts. And these guys were treating him day in, day out. They saw him at his worst. So, to then see him doing what he was doing and his recovery, I think that touched them as well. To actually think they had been part of that journey – to actually stop him from going." *John Price*

There were loads of people there. I did want to talk at length to them all but I just remember my wife had made this amazing soup and what I wanted to do most in that moment was eat! When you're attacking a challenge like the South Downs Way, a lot of what goes through your mind is when you're going to eat again. I was so hungry and I'd got so many people to talk to.

"We've got to get going soon," Tom said. "otherwise it'll be dark when we're getting in to Eastbourne."

I gulped down the soup, ate as much food as I could, said my farewells, then we set off again. The camera crew filmed us disappearing up the track away from Chantry Post car park along the South Downs Way, heading towards another epic climb ... Truleigh Hill.

To have the camaraderie of Tom and Mike on that ride meant a great deal. The banter throughout was good and we really needed it. As I'm sure many people who have done this ride will attest, it's hard work but especially hard work on your butt bones! About seventy-five to eighty miles in

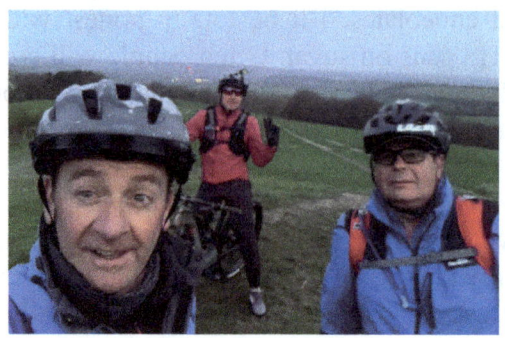

Figure 14

you start to really feel your legs complaining and the build-up of lactic acid in your muscles. The hills seem to keep coming, just as you are round the corner of a steep ascent ... oh, God, more!

Eventually though, there it was: a glimpse of the sea, peeking over the tops of the cliffs, along Beachy Head ... bloody hell, we'd nearly done it. Someone shot footage of us descending the steep downhill to the end (or start depending on how you look at it) of the South Downs Way at Eastbourne, so it could be sent off to the waiting team at ITV news, packaged up and aired along with the other film clips. It was a fantastic feeling to get to the end. Waiting there were my wife, daughters and a few friends. We'd made it! Feeling elated, tired and very pleased that it was over. I breathed a sigh of relief. What a journey! What a year.

We packed up our gear and Tom, Mike and I were driven back from Eastbourne. The return trip back was considerably quicker than the thirteen hours we'd just spent in the saddle. Stopping off in a village called Steyning, where there was a really nice chippy, we had a massive pile of fish and chips. We sat in the High Street, on the bonnet of the cars, eating our spoils, grinning at each other at what we'd achieved.

Tom looked at me, "Well done, mate. This time last year we thought you weren't going to make it out alive."

In that moment I was aware that I still had not fully comprehended what my body and mind had been through. This huge goal had given me an excuse to not think about the *what could have been*. It forced me to focus on getting fit and to giving myself a massive reason to get off my arse and *do*.

We went home to a hot shower and bed, I slept like a bloody log that night, no whirring machines keeping me alive, no false doors, no travelling bed, or desperate need to get home. I *was* home. I'd made it.

Chapter 29
Every end is a new beginning

The next day I watched the money coming in. Every minute: ding, ding, ding, ding. It was a euphoric moment. Originally, we set our sights on raising £5,000. We raised about £11,000 in the end. It's no Sir Tom but it was a good feeling.

I got messages from Luke Hodgson saying, "Bloody Hell, your step count was crazy!"

I had worn and was still wearing the Fitbit.

"I've never seen stats like this before," he added.

It really was a good feeling to have done it. We all felt really pleased to have accomplished the task. All that training had paid off. During the journey, I didn't reflect much on where I'd been a year before but people wouldn't let me forget, even if I wanted to. They kept saying, "F*** me. A year ago, you were nearly dead, mate. You're amazing."

But I didn't really feel amazing. The NHS is amazing. That was my go-to. This was my thank you to the NHS people, my attempt to shine a light on all that they had done for me … keeping me alive … on more than one occasion.

I'm sure it helped being internally driven, having goals, being willing to fight your inner demons, because the human psyche does have a predisposition towards, "Ah well, f*** it, I'll just stay in bed for another hour or I won't do it. I'll do it tomorrow in exchange for just another ten minutes under the warm, cosy duvet."

No, you need to do it now, because you've committed to doing it now. Training wasn't a piece of cake. I had to go

Every end is a new beginning

through that arduous process of: Oh, God, it's absolutely pissing with rain. I'm going to get wet. I'm going to get cold. It's going to be horrible. My left foot and leg were still not a hundred per cent and often times my right leg felt like it was doing more of the work but I HAVE to do it. I'm choosing to do it and I know why.

As part of my training, I remember cycling up to the top of the South Downs one morning in February. It was so icy cold that there were these amazing vertical icicles that were hanging off the fencing where it had rained and then, being blown one way, had frozen. There was crunchy frost everywhere because we used to get out early. You were out there for a good three, four, five hours, bashing the bike, making a beeline for some cafe somewhere so you could get a greasy sausage roll and coffee. So, you could try and defrost your toes and fingers before heading towards home.

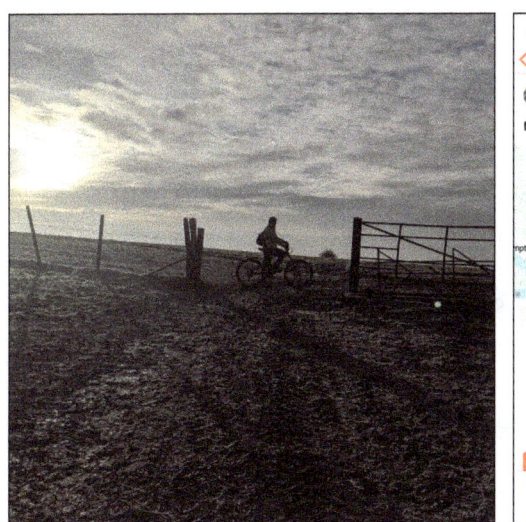
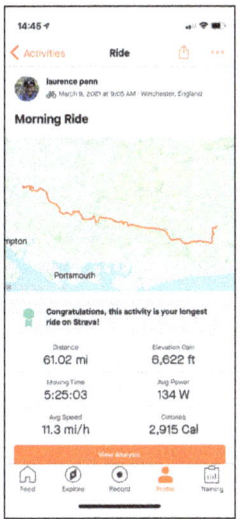

Figure 15   *Figure 16*

There were a few lovely mornings but most of the time it would just be wet and windy. It was often absolutely pissing with rain because it's Great Britain after all. It all needed to be accepted. Whatever the weather, I was all in. I just thank God it wasn't wet and windy on the day of doing the big ride. It was fantastic because we were in t-shirts at some stages.

Maybe that was a lesson I had to hang on to? To hang on for the light because there's going to be dark, hard times and in those times, you learn a lot about yourself. Having COVID-19 has absolutely, fundamentally changed my life completely. I wouldn't wish it on anyone, not having COVID-19 or being that ill, but it certainly underlines this: you only live once.

That expression … *You only live once*. Well, it's wrong. You only die once. You live every single day, so make the most of it. That became my mantra of a sort. And then Tom used to say, "Mate, we're here for a good time not a long time." If you want to allow negativity to take hold, you go for it. If you want to stay positive, choose that direction. Sometimes, it's as easy as that. Making the choice. Then the hard work can start.

You decide what story you're going to believe about what you're capable of. If you've been unwell and suffered and made the choice today to walk one mile where you know you were capable of walking ten miles before, you'll be able to do it if you keep this mental fortitude and keep telling yourself, yes, I can do this. There are so many excuses that your brain makes on the way: choosing comfort, the easy option. I think we're programmed to be comfortable. Push through the comfort, discipline comes before motivation.

Contrary to some of the comments I've received, I suppose I don't see myself as any kind of superhero. I'm not. However, I would love to help other people tune into that frequency of the brain and the way it works. And if they've been unfortunate enough to spend time in ICU or been gravely ill, for whatever reason, to know there is a path they could follow with some proven results backed by statistics from brilliant research using a smartwatch and championed by Drs Hodgson and Leckie. It's going to be hard, but anything in life worth having is. There's always a bit of grit needed.

I asked some members of the physiotherapist team that assisted me through this extraordinary time in my life, what factors seemed to really help with a successful recovery after a stay on ICU. Gemma Stoner said, "Motivation, that's an obvious one. People who are motivated and positive tend to do well."

Fellow physio Mary-Kate Standing added, "And they see this as an opportunity to turn their lives around. This has been a reality check of sorts. It changes their outlook on life."

The physios said some people come back to the clinic and actually say that they are fitter and happier now than before they went into ICU.

"I think the fact they leave hospital and then they know that they're going to get followed up in three months, it puts that ownership on them. They know we're tracking them, plus the motivation we give, like the goal setting, I think is a huge factor as well. I think we are there for the majority of their journey in the hospital. Obviously, when they first come on to ICU, we're seeing them when they're extremely unwell and they're on a ventilator. Then we're the first ones that start getting them moving, then they're going down to the wards and seeing more physios, or one of us again. We're there throughout their journey and get to know them really well, which I think plays a huge part in their recovery." *Jessica Owen*

Amelia Palmer said, "I think family and friends maybe as well. It can be really helpful motivation, whether it's that their family and friends are supportive or that they encourage them, whether it's that they even enable them in like, oh they can come to the clinic or they can go to the gym because they've got someone who can take them. But also, as a motivation, some people say: I need to get better for my grandchildren; I want to still be able to play with them; or, I need to get better so I can help my wife because she's not very well herself. So, it's important I'm well enough to do it. I think, having that sort of life purpose as well as support that comes from family and friends." *Amelia Palmer*

*

Having COVID-19 led me to reassess my lifestyle. I don't work like I used to. I gave a lot of it up. I'm very fortunate with the company I was employed with prior to and during COVID-19 and I think they could see that I wasn't going to come back. We architected a situation where I could resign. They paid me very well for doing that. I had to sign a one year non-compete, so I couldn't go after their clients. The CEO was very generous and I'm very grateful for his support.

I took all that time off to reinvent myself, get fit and strong again and not fall into old habits, to walk the walk, to jettison useless habits and toxic relationships. I reduced the amount I was travelling right down. No more being in so many cars, trains and planes. No more three-hour daily commutes.

I checked in with myself (at the suggestion of my good friend, Tom), asked myself much more often: Do I really want to be doing this? That was huge.

There were lots of defining, changing moments and there

came a point where I realised the fairy tale would stop soon because I needed to earn money. I was being approached but I knew I didn't want to find just another company to join, another boardroom to frequent, I'm a self–starter. I got this.

Thankfully, the business I set up is going well. I work from home. I've been to London a handful of times in the last few years. Whereas, before COVID-19, I'd be there twenty times a month, because that's where it was happening and that was where you had to be, right? Turns out that was partly nonsense. You don't.

So many of my dreams when I was in that coma were about trying to be somewhere else, but it turned out the place I wanted to be wasn't Dubai, Baltimore or London. It wasn't exotic or high flying or even where the party was. It was domestic. It was home. It was a hug.

Mischa added to this sentiment, "I will say that my dad continues to amaze me with how strong he is, how persistent he is. He'll act like nothing happened. He'll act like it was just a short, weak cold. I think for him, having COVID-19 definitely kind of shook him a little bit. It woke him up to say, f*** it, life's too short. Don't let people control you. Do what you want to do. Money … should it be an object? Well, it shouldn't be, so don't let it control you.

I feel like I see a connection between my mum and dad that I didn't see before and I think it's both of them appreciating the fact that they've got a really sweet life together. A life together they might not have had. My mum appreciates turning a dark event into a light event. I think we both value going through it because it makes you grateful for your family, grateful for your position and it obviously makes you grateful for the fact that you've come out the other end.

Dad's definitely shifted. I think Mum's shifted as well.

I can see that they are much more connected now, which is really lovely to see. Dad's also changed his mindset. He doesn't let a lot of things stop him. They're living their life a lot more, which I really appreciate. I will say, off the back of it, they've become people I aspire to be." *Mischa Penn*

*

I think the world has changed a lot around where you work and maybe even what work is really about. Some of the work people do is much more about their output than the destination of the output. I know companies in London where they've got office space for a hundred people and they've only got thirty people attending the office because everyone went home, worked from home and they don't want to come back. They don't want to spend six grand a year on a season ticket to sit on a train. They're saving six grand. They're seeing more of their wife or their husband or their kids or they're going to the gym or walking the dog, creating better habits. Realising that they are important – health is important ... So, why would they want to flee back into London or to commuting in general? The tech is there, so let's use it.

I see the struggle that companies have going on right now, because they think it's going to dilute their culture. Whereas, I think, if you allow people to work in this new way, you'll develop a better, stronger culture built around trust. Companies can really benefit from building that trust. If your team can be trusted to deliver what you need to be delivered and jump on a video call, it can really work wonders.

I studied Neuro-Linguistic Programming (NLP) years ago with Paul McKenna, because I was fascinated to understand human communication, not just verbal, but all the cues. I wanted to understand body language, the words and actions we use to describe a certain situation. It's served me incredibly well in breaking down hostile situations with people, quickly getting on to their wavelength, using their body language, using the words they're using, getting them to think differently. Therefore, I do totally value face-to-face time. It's the ultimate communication. That means when you do a Zoom call, you are losing some of it, but if it's just to say: OK, well, here are the numbers. Or, this is where we are to target, etcetera. Do you really need to travel hours to see someone for that?

If you're going to go and try and win a £5 million deal or something, I think you've got to invest some actual face-to-face time in that, but as for trudging from Slough to London every day just because the boss wants you there, I think that's prehistoric. It's not the way forward. Certainly, it doesn't fit with the environment, or the desperate need to cut down on fuel and wasted journeys.

The experience I had changed my values. Not only did I develop a new sense of worth in my home, myself, my relationship with my wife, but also in my relationship with planet earth. It forced me to stop and smell the roses, to reassess. A lot of stuff I worried about before is now gone. I just let it go: anger, resentment, stress and worry. It doesn't burden me anymore. In fact, you can only deal with what's in front of you, worrying is an absolute waste of time.

*

Dr Tim Fooks added, "Anybody who does a role like mine, where you become empathetic, it's a great joy to see someone who was taken to the very edge of life, to being cared for in such a way that he's actually managed to get better. But then to see someone like Laurence, who's taken that in such a constructive way, and is obviously being as proactively positive as he can be, is amazing. And I think that sort of resilience and courage ... it's nice to stand alongside, isn't it? The phrase: it's a warm glow on a cold morning, is a nice way to think of it.

I think, sadly, you have to accept in my work that not everybody recovers and you can't go around feeling that you're somehow to blame for people not getting better. But it's lovely to be any part of someone's journey where they've gone through the ringer and have come out the other side. So, yeah, he's an even more special person than he was before, put it that way. Keeping ourselves fit and well is like keeping a healthy bank balance. You've got the resources to draw on when you go through a real hard time and he's a good example of why that's important." *Dr Tim Fooks*

*

I asked Martine to sum up her awful experience, "... through it all, the waiting, the fear, the endless uncertainty, I was carrying something so heavy I could barely name it. I lived in a kind of suspended state, bracing for every phone call, never knowing if it would bring good news, bad news, or no change at all. There were no clear answers, no guarantees. Just love, and the sheer determination to keep going.

I was coping the only way I knew how: moment by moment. Some days I was strong, some days I was barely holding it together. But I kept showing up. I became the calm voice for Loz when he was scared and confused. Even when I was terrified myself. I held it together for him, because I had to. He needed an anchor and I did my best to be that – even when I felt like I was drowning.

There were moments that softened the edges, the nurses who took the time to speak to me in the garden, the warmth of Gemma asking to know who Loz really was. That conversation meant so much. Being asked about him not as a patient, but as a person. As my person. It reminded me that love and care can still reach through PPE and fear and hospital walls.

I was scared, often overwhelmed, but I never stopped loving him fiercely. I never stopped hoping. I didn't have training for this. I didn't have a guidebook. But I kept going. I gave it everything I had. I was strong, not because I wasn't afraid, but because I kept moving forward in spite of that fear. That's how I coped. That's how I survived." *Martine Penn*

*

I'm not advocating people have a spell in ICU to get here. However, there are ways to think and feel differently. For me, it started with really wanting to help people, most especially the people who had, under the most extraordinary circumstances, helped me. I wanted to help the NHS. I wanted to help Dr Hodgson with the Fitbit project and to hopefully get them into every ICU department in the country. Helping became a way of fighting off feelings of despair. It gave me purpose.

I could have easily parked up Self Pity Lane and stayed there if I didn't have anyone checking in on me. You can say, "I'll do that tomorrow," and then tomorrow becomes next week, becomes next month ... It doesn't happen. Then you get depressed and you get annoyed with yourself. That's the root. The horrible spinning cycle of self-loathing and it leads to anxiety because I haven't done what I needed to do.

Anybody who works in the NHS will want to keep people out of hospital and the root to that is better health, better mental health, better physical health, a better version of you. And it can be achieved no matter how hard it might be. I understand how all that happens. I really do.

My foot still isn't a hundred per cent and I can definitely feel my lungs have less capacity due to the scarring but my mind is sharp and my self-belief is high. I believe the mind is the muscle we ultimately have to work on the most ... those guys at Nike were on to something when they said: *Just do it*.

Appendices – The clinical view of events and some data provided by the NHS

Date	Treatment
30th March 2020	admission overnight into CPAP hood, Fibrinogen 9
31st March 2020	intubated overnight due to increasing respiratory failure
1st April 2020	settled Fi02 045 on recovery trial (usual care)
2nd April 2020	IPPV continued, Trop <10
2nd April 2020	Dalteparin--> bd as felt to be prothrombotic
3rd April 2020	O2 requirement reduced – fiO2 40 LFTs up: proned
4th April 2020	second prone in the eve; reducing fiO2 overnight
5th April 2020	supinated@1300 third prone in eve
6th April 2020	supinated. Hb drop, switch from Ranitidine to Omeprazole
7th April 2020	BNO for NG water
8th April 2020	worsening ventilation with associated worsening changes on CXR
9th April 2020	APRV started in evening/ night
10th April 2020	uraemia improving may still need filter; new CVC and art line
11th April 2020	4th prone
14th April 2020	proned 5th time

15th April 2020	proned again overnight 6th time
16th April 2020	consider trache[ostomy] when ventilation improves
17th April 2020	sedation hold. Discuss trache[ostomy] with ENT, Sat? Mon?
18th April 2020	surgical trache[ostomy] (adjustable flange size 9) NO INNER CANNULA started on methylpred[nisolone]
19th April 2020	stable
20th April 2020	stable
21st April 2020	weaning sedation
22nd April 2020	stable on weaning plan
23rd April 2020	stop sedation, continue wean
24th April 2020	ongoing T wean 2 units RBC
25th April 2020	ongoing T wean slept well
26th April 2020	good spirits
27th April 2020	trial of speaking valve
28th April 2020	progressing well with wean
29th April 2020	twenty-four hours on trache[ostomy] mask. Cognition improving but tires easily
30th April 2020	trache[ostomy] decannulated
1st May 2020	strength of voice not improving, discussed with SALT
2nd May 2020	steadily improving
3rd May 2020	wearable (Fitbit) improving remains tachycardic
4th May 2020	suitable for ward step down

Days ventilated – 29

GP information – discharge from ICU

Patients who have a had a long stay on ICU (usually over three days ventilation) often require additional organ support as well as long periods of immobility and sedation. As a result, they may experience long-term post-intensive care syndrome (PICS) such as:

- Musculoskeletal – critical illness polyneuropathy (CIPNM) muscle weakness, pain, falls
- Psychological – anxiety, depression, cognitive dysfunction, PTSD: nightmares, hallucinations and flashbacks
- Oropharyngeal – dysphagia and malnutrition, weight loss, change to normal bowel habit

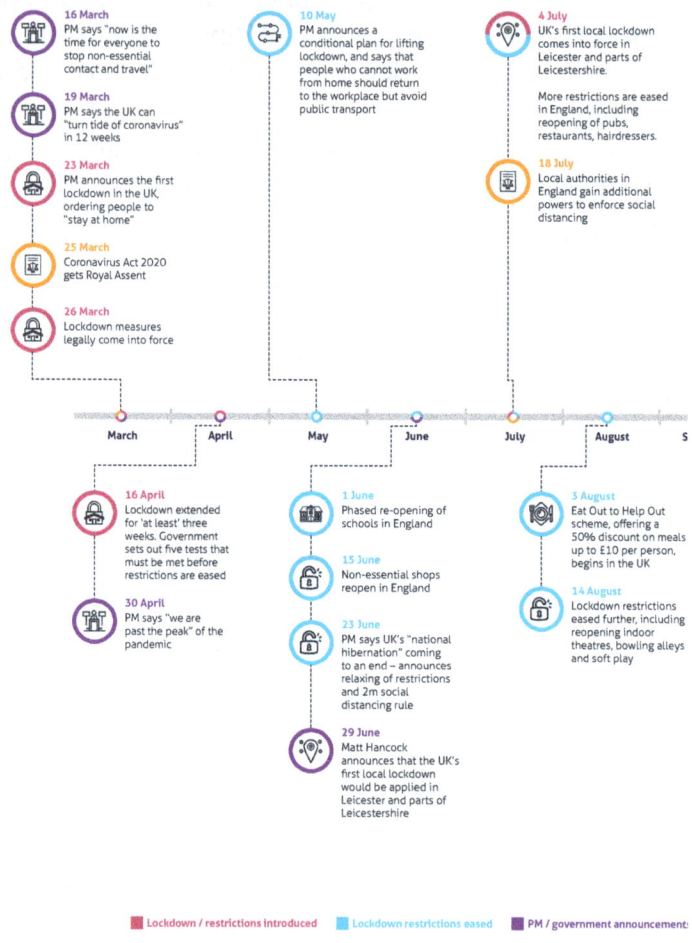

Source: Institute for Government analysis.

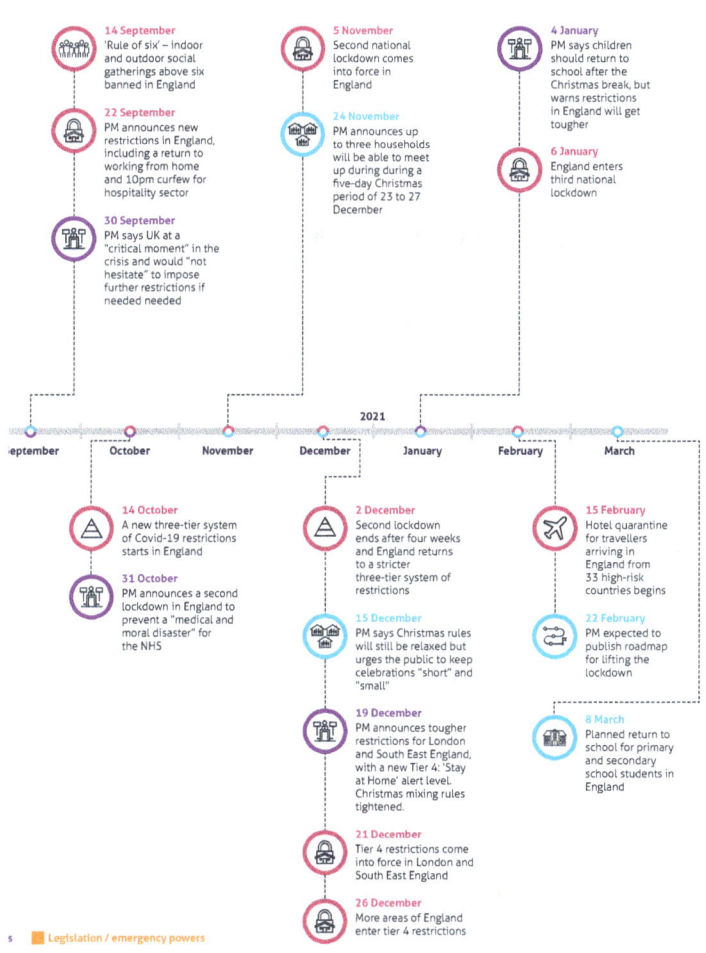

List of Images

All images are the Penn family's own, apart from figures 4 and 5 – see citations.

Page vii	Fig 1	Thanks and acknowledgements: the A Team: Amelia Palmer, Dr Luke Hodgson, Dr Todd Leckie, Mary-Kate Standing
Page 31	Fig 2	The next thing I knew, I was wearing what appeared to be a dated spaceman's helmet. It went over my entire head and round my shoulders. The device was pumping out a hundred per cent oxygen in a desperate attempt to get it into my blood stream.
Page 33	Fig 3	My hospital admission notes show that on the 28th of March 2020 at 21:23, a fifty–four-year-old man was officially admitted to Worthing Hospital. He had a severely low oxygen count, shortness of breath, a high fever and a cough. He was otherwise an extremely fit, active man. Just over twenty-four hours later he was admitted to ICU as his condition declined.

Page 63	Fig 4		Nurses wore masks and full PPE for at least three hours, until having a break. Marks appeared on their faces and their skin was affected.
Page 68	Fig 5		With me being flat out on the bed, the risk of pressure sores where infections might occur is a concern. The team have to keep all the plates spinning. The battle for my life was not about beating just COVID-19 itself but all the chaos it had created.
Page 90	Fig 6		"… I actually started the steroids on him that evening when he was still pretty static and there was quite a dramatic improvement over time to that. And certainly that CRP just shot down. Obviously – you could say – was it doing the tracheostomy that was partly helpful as well, but his lung function essentially just started to improve."
Page 123	Fig 7		The first time I stood up again was daunting. With no balance, no strength, someone was holding each of my arms for support. After that came walking with a frame with a physio either side of me and one behind.

Page 175   Fig 8   We just sat there having a gin and tonic and reflecting over what we had been through. I looked out over the amazing scenery and thought, thank God. Thank God this turned out the way it did. Looking back now, Cornwall was where I turned a corner.

Page 185   Fig 9   They put me on an exercise bike, strangely enough, strapped up with heart monitors, a breath monitor, and then, "Every minute," they said, "We're going to increase the resistance on the bike. You can't stand up, so you have to stay sitting down and just go for it."

Page 187   Fig 10   I was almost like a 360-degree: This guy's bounced back! It made me all the more determined to raise money for the NHS with my epic bike ride. I had to make them proud

Page 187   Fig 11   Two guys from ITV Meridian turned up, an interviewer, Malcolm Shaw and a cameraman. We had a conversation. They came to our house and filmed a piece. During the filming we arranged to link up with Amelia Palmer live on a Zoom call. Getting it aired on ITV was pretty daunting.

List of Images

Page 198   Fig 12   Through being a research champion, I got another unique invitation. Out of the blue, I was asked to be a judge for the *Nursing Times* Awards

Page 201   Fig 13   We stopped roughly every twenty to twenty-five miles to refuel, keeping up the calories before we cracked on again. About fifty to fifty-five miles in, Storrington marked the halfway point.

Page 204   Fig 14   To have the camaraderie of Tom and Mike on that ride meant a great deal.

Page207   Fig 15   I remember cycling up to the top of the South Downs one morning in February. It was so icy cold that there were these amazing vertical icicles that were hanging off the fencing where it had rained and then, being blown one way, had frozen. There was crunchy frost everywhere because we used to get out early.

Page 207   Fig 16   You were out there for a good three, four, five hours, bashing the bike, making a beeline for some cafe somewhere so you could get a greasy sausage roll and coffee. So, you could try and defrost your toes and fingers before heading towards home.

Glossary

All references include NHS terminology to medically and accurately explain the terms.

Name	Description
44th Dimbleby Lecture	Professor Dame Sarah Gilbert delivers an account of the development of the Oxford AstraZeneca Covid-19 vaccine, which has now been used in more than 170 countries.
Arrhythmias	Heart rhythm problems (arrhythmia) are when your heart beats too quickly or too slowly or your heartbeat is not steady.
ARDS – see also proning	Acute respiratory distress syndrome – Acute respiratory distress syndrome (ARDS) is a life-threatening illness that can happen when your lungs are not working properly. ARDS is usually a complication of other serious conditions and is treated in hospital.

Glossary

Blood gas tests	Blood gas analysis involves measuring the levels of oxygen (O2), carbon dioxide (CO2), and pH in the blood, as well as other parameters such as bicarbonate (HCO3-) and oxygen saturation (SaO2).
Butterfly effect	The butterfly effect is a theory that small changes can lead to big consequences over time. It's a concept in chaos theory that's often used in popular culture.
Clap for the NHS	The weekly clapping for NHS staff and other key workers ran for 10 weeks during the first coronavirus lockdown, under the name Clap for Our Carers.
TCRNCC	Clinical Research Network Coordinating Centre is a service provided by the Consortium, supported by a wider partnership which includes King's College London, Imperial College London, Newcastle University, University of Liverpool and PA Consulting Services Limited

	The CRNCC manages the NIHR Clinical Research Network ("CRN") on behalf of the Department of Health and Social Care. The CRN makes it possible for patients and health professionals across England to participate in clinical research studies within the NHS.
Comorbidity	Comorbidity simply means more than one illness or disease occurring in one person at the same time and multimorbidity means more than two illnesses or diseases occurring in the same person at the same time.
Convalescent Plasma	The convalescent plasma treatment in this trial was for people who had been in intensive care for less than 48 hours and have tested positive for COVID-19. People who received plasma as part of their treatment had two transfusions over two days and were monitored for 21 days to see how effective this was.

Glossary

                              The trial paused enrolment for patients in intensive care in January 2021 and began to analyse the data.
The initial analysis of all trial patients requiring intensive care unit support showed that convalescent plasma did not improve outcomes. The final analysis is in progress and the results of this are awaited.

CUE-TIP	Covid-19 Understanding and Elimination–Trials Implementation Panel
CRP Levels and Covid-19	C-reactive protein (CRP) is a non-specific acute phase reactant elevated in infection or inflammation. Higher levels indicate more severe infection and have been used as an indicator of COVID-19 disease severity. When Laurence would have been hospitalised CRP responses in patients hospitalised with COVID-19 were used to determine the utility of CRP on admission for predicting inpatient mortality.

BED NO. 1

Dexamethasone	Dexamethasone tablets and liquid Brand names: Neofordex, Glensoludex, Martapan. Dexamethasone tablets and liquid treat inflammatory conditions and autoimmune conditions.
ENT	Ear, nose, and throat (ENT) NHS services diagnose and treat conditions affecting the head and neck. This includes the ears, nose, throat, mouth, face, salivary glands, and thyroid gland.
Genomic	Genomics is the study of the genes in our DNA, their functions and their influence on the growth, development and working of the body – using a variety of techniques to look at the body's DNA and associated compounds.
HDU	High dependency unit – The High Dependency Unit sits within the Critical Care Department next to Intensive Care.

Glossary

Hydroxychloroquine	From March 1 to April 30, 2020, Donald J Trump made 11 tweets about unproven therapies and mentioned these therapies 65 times in White House briefings, especially touting hydroxychloroquine and chloroquine. The drugs did not help coronavirus patients, and should not be used outside clinical trials, researchers said. An analysis of 96,000 patients shows those treated with hydroxychloroquine were also more likely to suffer irregular heart rhythms.
ITU – also known as ICU	Intensive therapy unit, also known as intensive care unit – intensive therapy is a branch of medicine concerned with the diagnosis and management of life-threatening conditions. Patients in intensive therapy require close monitoring and support from equipment and medication to keep normal body functions going.

They may be unable to breathe on their own and have multiple organ failure. This type of care cannot be provided on a typical ward, as highly specialised devices are required, along with the personnel who are trained to use it safely.

Iatrogenic harms — Iatrogenesis refers to harm experienced by patients resulting from medical care, whereas negligence is more narrowly conceived as deviation from standard care.

ISARIC — The International Severe Acute Respiratory and emerging Infection Consortium (ISARIC) is a global federation of investigator-led clinical research networks: a network of networks. ISARIC has over sixty member networks, and many partners, from around the world. Together we conduct clinical research to improve patients' care and facilitate a globally coordinated and agile research response to infectious disease threats.

	For over a decade, we have been generating clinically meaningful research evidence for diseases including COVID-19, dengue, Ebola, Lassa fever, Nipah, mpox and bubonic plague.
Methylprednisolone	Steroids, also called corticosteroids, are anti-inflammatory medicines used to treat a range of conditions.
Sir Tom Moore	Captain Sir Thomas Moore, more popularly known as Captain Tom, was a British Army officer and fundraiser. He made international headlines in April 2020 when he raised money for charity in the run-up to his 100th birthday during the COVID-19 pandemic.
MDT	A multidisciplinary team is a group of health and care staff who are members of different organisations and professions (e.g. GPs, social workers, nurses), that work together to make decisions regarding the treatment of individual patients and service users. MDTs are used in both health and care settings.

NIHR	National Institute for Health and Care Research is committed to funding health, public health and social care research that leads to improved outcomes for patients and the public, and makes the health and social care system more efficient, effective and safe.
NLP	Neuro-Linguistic Programming is a method of communication and personal development that focuses on how language, feelings, and thoughts are organised. It's based on the idea that people have internal maps of the world that are shaped by their sensory experience
PPEI	Patient and Public Engagement and Involvement was introduced following the Health and Social Care Act 2012 introduced significant amendments to the NHS Act 2006.

Glossary

	Specifically, it introduced two new legal duties, requiring Clinical Commissioning Groups (CCGs) and commissioners in NHS England to enable: patients and carers to participate in planning, managing and making decisions about their care and treatment, through the services they commission; the effective participation of the public in the commissioning process itself, so that services provided reflect the needs of local people.
PPE	Personal protective equipment is most commonly used by nursing staff includes gloves, aprons and respiratory protective equipment (RPE) such as FFP3 masks.
Proning	Proning is a treatment technique used for patients with acute respiratory distress syndrome (ARDS) where the patient is positioned on their stomach (prone position) instead of their back (supine position).

	This helps improve oxygenation by redistributing air and blood flow more evenly throughout the lungs, potentially leading to better gas exchange and improved breathing function in severe cases of ARDS; this is considered a standard of care for patients with severe ARDS requiring mechanical ventilation.
SALT team or SLT	The speech and language therapy team help patients with speech, communication, and swallowing needs, predominantly of neurological or structural origin. They help people with a range of conditions, including head injuries, neurosurgical and neurodegenerative disorders like dementia, Huntington's disease, motor neurone disease, Parkinson's disease, progressive supranuclear palsy and multiple system atrophy.

Tracheostomy	A tracheostomy (also called a tracheotomy) is a procedure where a hole is made at the front of the neck. A tube is inserted through the opening and into the windpipe (trachea) to help you breathe.
Reasons you may need to have a tracheostomy include:
to help you breathe if your throat is blocked
to remove excess fluid and mucus from your lungs
to deliver oxygen from a machine called a ventilator to your lungs
A tracheostomy is often planned in advance, but sometimes it needs to be done as soon as possible in an emergency.
If you need a tracheostomy but are unable to give your consent, it will be discussed with your family.

University of Oxford's Recovery Trial	RECOVERY started in the UK in early 2020 as the Randomised Evaluation of COVID-19 Therapy, a clinical trial testing treatments for people admitted to hospital with COVID-19 pneumonia. One trial. Over 47,000 participants. Nearly 200 hospital sites, across six countries. Ten results. Four effective COVID-19 treatments. And behind them all, an army of countless researchers, doctors, nurses, statisticians and supporting staff.
WHO	World Health Organisation – The World Health Organization is a specialised agency of the United Nations responsible for global public health. It is headquartered in Geneva, Switzerland, and has six regional offices and 150 field offices worldwide.

About the Author

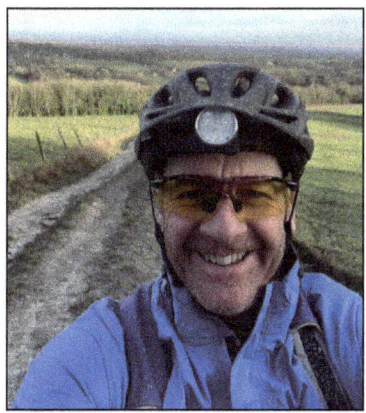

Laurence Penn lives in a West Sussex village, called Thakeham. He has worked within the IT professional and IT managed services industry setting up the supply of in demand IT resources to projects across the globe for large multinational businesses. Developing and running sales and delivery teams in UK, Europe, South Africa, Asia and the middle east would see him often travelling frequently. These projects often utilised teams of 200 plus specialist contractors.

Laurence is also a father of two daughters and his wife, Martine, is a keen equestrian and they have land to keep horses and make hay. In his spare time, he has always had many hobbies that keep him fit and active, from jiu-jitsu, mountain biking, squash, badminton, padel tennis, fitness training and sailing/ boating.

During the period when the book is set, Laurence was working with a consulting business, turning round sales and operations functions. He was about eighteen months into the role when COVID-19 hit ...

Notes on contributors

Grace Dowding	Neurological Physiotherapist a former Recruiter from Brighton, moved into the NHS eight years ago.
Linda Folkes	Public Research Champion at University Hospitals Sussex NHS Foundation Trust, now retired from a stunning forty-two-year career with the NHS majoring in Dermatology.
Heather Fox	Registered Nurse at University Hospitals Sussex, working within cardiology, ICU and Research.
Tim Fooks (Dr)	High Sheriff of West Sussex and former general practice owner, Tim sits on the Board and Education Committee of the Leathersellers' Livery Company in the City of London and is a trustee and patron to several West Sussex charities and an experienced sailor.
Luke Hodgson (Dr)	Intensive Care and Respiratory Consultant at University Hospitals Sussex NHS Foundation Trust, Honorary Clinical Reader at BSMS, with an interest in applied technology in acute care settings.

Notes on contributors

Todd Leckie (Dr)	Anaesthetics and intensive care medicine doctor. Prior to starting work as a doctor, he competed internationally as a triathlete and represented Great Britain at World Championship level.
Sam Morfee	Staff Nurse at Western Sussex Hospitals NHS Trust, also a rather brilliant golfer.
Amelia Palmer	Respiratory Network Manager at NHS Sussex and a keen distance runner.
Martine Penn	Laurence's wife, degree qualified finance professional now retrained as an equine assisted psychotherapist. Keen equestrian.
Mischa Penn	Laurence's daughter, working in IT providing cloud-based solutions with Azure, Google Cloud and Amazon Web Services.
Jessica Owen	Department of Physiotherapy.
John Price	Charity Ambassador for My University Hospitals Sussex and supporting the NHS for eleven years.
Tom Simmonds	Laurence's friend who supported his training and journey on the South Downs Way in one day. Tom runs a successful business within the fire safety industry and is revolutionising using software in this space.

BED NO. 1

Mary-Kate Standing	Senior Respiratory Physiotherapist.
Gemma Stoner	Department of Physiotherapy.
Mike Wood	School Friend, South Downs Way in a day and training buddy.

One last thing before you go ...

Dear reader,

I hope you've enjoyed Bed Number One and will add your review to Amazon, Goodreads and to your social media platforms. Please share my book's cover with your social media review.

Thank you so much for reading my story and those of my family and my NHS family.

Best wishes,

Laurence Penn
Laurence Penn

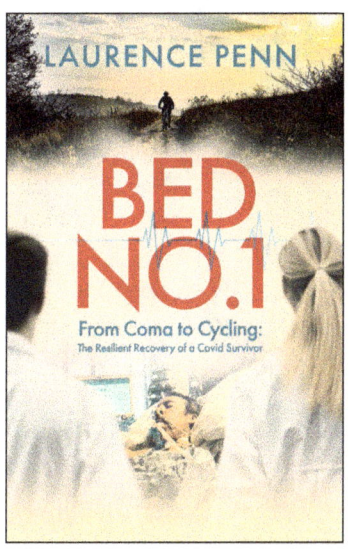

Bed Number One – fundraising

For news about my fundraising via sales of this book and the work of John Price and his team for My University Hospitals Sussex, please follow my website:

www.bednumberone.com

Or follow this QRcode to my website:

Best wishes,
Laurence Penn
Laurence Penn

BED NO. 1

www.ingramcontent.com/pod-product-compliance
Lightning Source LLC
Chambersburg PA
CBHW051537020426
42333CB00016B/1971